To Your Health

Helena Chmura Kraemer

Karen Kraemer Lowe

David J. Kupfer

To Your Health

How to Understand What Research Tells Us About Risk

OXFORD
UNIVERSITY PRESS

2005

OXFORD
UNIVERSITY PRESS

Oxford University Press, Inc., publishes works that further
Oxford University's objective of excellence
in research, scholarship, and education.

Oxford New York
Auckland Cape Town Dar es Salaam Delhi Hong Kong Karachi
Kuala Lumpur Madrid Melbourne Mexico City Nairobi
New Delhi Shanghai Taipei Toronto

With offices in
Argentina Austria Brazil Chile Czech Republic France Greece
Guatemala Hungary Italy Japan Poland Portugal Singapore
South Korea Switzerland Thailand Turkey Ukraine Vietnam

Published by Oxford University Press, Inc.
198 Madison Avenue, New York, New York 10016

www.oup.com

Library of Congress Cataloging-in-Publication Data
Kraemer, Helena Chmura.
To your health : how to understand what research tells us about risk / by
Helena Chmura Kraemer, Karen Kraemer Lowe, and David J. Kupfer.
p. cm.
Includes bibliographical references and index.
ISBN-13 978-0-19-517870-8
ISBN 0-19-517870-X
1. Health risk assessment. 2. Self-care, Health. I. Lowe, Karen
Kraemer. II. Kupfer, David J., 1941–III. Title.
RA427 .3. K73 2005
613—dc22 2004017721

9 8 7 6 5 4 3 2 1

Printed in the United States of America
on acid-free paper

We dedicate this book to the memory of David (Dan) Offord, who exemplified the highest commitment to his patients while demonstrating how scientific ability and rigor could push the boundaries of improved clinical care.

Preface

Over the 40-plus years of our careers in psychiatry, medicine, and biostatistics, we have seen many advances in science, research methods, computing, and analysis capabilities. Yet even today, little is known of the etiology of most psychiatric disorders and very little is known about their prevention, early identification, or cure. We know risk factors, and we have treatment options, but fundamentally, many of the most life-disrupting psychiatric disorders continue to be diagnosed at rates higher than, or just as high as, when we began our careers.

Two of us (H.C.K. and D.J.K.) have collaborated for the past 20 years addressing these issues in two MacArthur Foundation research networks—one on depression and the other on psychopathology and development. Despite our different backgrounds, we have sought common ground to improve the level of communication in our field by insisting on precise terminology. A series of publications involving risk research, written together with many of our MacArthur network colleagues, represented the fruits of these efforts.

In that process, we began to appreciate the need for clearer communication across disciplines, among and between scientists and clinicians, and between clinicians and "consumers of medical and health information"—patients, family members, and policy makers. We were having trouble recommending the best articles in behavioral research to document all the interesting advances in psychiatry. But we quickly realized that these difficulties were not limited to behavioral research, but rather were present throughout medicine and health communication.

Besides, in addition to being academics and researchers, we too are "medical consumers"—individuals who strive to improve our own health and the health of our families. With our extensive medical and statistical training, we too couldn't make heads or tails of some of the advice about what puts us at risk for certain diseases or disorders and how we can prevent them. Many of the examples we have used in this book touch each of us personally—the prostate-specific antigen (PSA) test, hormone replacement therapy (HRT), mammography, and topics concerning young children, including television watching, sleep, breast-feeding, and attention disorders.

We have observed a lack of accurate information, with much of that information being overinterpreted, overstated, conflicting, or confusing. Yet this is the same information being used to guide medical decisions for ourselves, our families, and our communities. Thus, we strove to write a book that was intended to address more than just researchers and students. Instead, this book is meant to provide tools to help all who are looking for credible information about health and disease. As we write in late 2004, well into the incredible genetics, neuroscience, and information technology revolutions, we are optimistic that the essential tools we provide here to access these advances will be employed by all who hope to improve their health and the quality of their lives.

We are grateful to the John D. and Catherine T. MacArthur Foundation in Chicago for support provided to this initiative through the Research Network on Psychopathology and Development (David J. Kupfer, M.D., Network Chair). In addition to financial support, we are indebted to the MacArthur Foundation for the vision shown in creating a mechanism of support to foster the process of intellectual networking across disciplines and fields and to encourage the out-of-the-box thinking required to solve complex research problems. Many of us who have been privileged to participate in MacArthur research networks have been profoundly affected by the collaborative and transdisciplinary experience afforded in these settings, and the concept has since been emulated and accepted as a "best practice" for pushing difficult fields and issues toward more rapid progress.

Hermi Rojahn Woodward was the administrator for both those networks, and both her contributions to organization of our work and travel and her direct contributions to the discussions of such issues cannot be overestimated or overappreciated.

The earliest roots for this book date back to discussions among colleagues within the MacArthur Research Network on Psychopathology and

Development about potential reasons for slow progress toward elucidating the etiology of mental health problems in childhood and adolescence. Through these discussions, several network members stimulated the formulation of more precise terminology to define risk-related terms, critiqued emerging concepts, and participated as coauthors in the earliest peer-reviewed publications to advance standardized terminology and improved methods for identifying risk factors. Our sincere thanks to our colleagues Alan Kazdin, Peter Jensen, and Ron Kessler for their contributions to the earlier phases of this work. The late Dan Offord infused our efforts with meaning by highlighting, again and again, the importance of improved risk factor identification for the development of interventions to reduce the burden of suffering incurred by children and adolescents with mental health problems and their families. We thank our colleague Tom Boyce for his many contributions to conceptual discussions during the later phases of this work. Finally, we are deeply indebted to our colleague Marilyn Essex, who courageously agreed to let us test many of the emerging concepts in her large longitudinal data set, the Wisconsin Study of Family and Work. Throughout the years, her continued enthusiasm for our collaborative work and her good humor in the face of laborious data-analytic endeavors have been an inspiration to all of us.

The other members of the network provided an extraordinarily receptive and critical audience for our efforts, allowing us to try out our ideas and providing us a sharp edge against which to hone those ideas: Floyd Bloom, Ron Dahl, Ellen Frank, the late Richard Harrington, Dan Keating, Ann Masten, Kathy Merikangas, Chuck Nelson, and Larry Steinberg.

We particularly thank Jerry Yesavage, who showed an early and consistent interest in considering with us the clinical and research implications of these methods and in trying them out and, even more important, who spent his vacation programming the public access software that is used here and is available to all readers to implement the ROC tree method. At the University of Pittsburgh, we thank John Scott, who programmed the software used here to implement the moderator–mediator analyses. Without these resources, many of the approaches would remain of theoretical interest but unavailable for anyone other than truly dedicated specialists.

In addition, many researchers, more than we could possibly name individually, provided us an ongoing sounding board for our ideas, and, even more important, provided us the opportunity to apply these ideas in their very diverse research projects: the MTA Cooperative Group in its study of effectiveness of treatment of attention-deficit/hyperactivity disorder, especially Jim Swanson and Steve Hinshaw; Drs. W. Stewart Agras, Terry Wilson, Tim Walsh, and Chris Fairburn in their multicenter study of treatment for bulimia; investigators at the Stanford Center for Research into Disease

Prevention, especially Marilyn Winkleby, Michaela Kiernan, Abby King, Joel Killen, and Tom Robinson; and investigators at the Stanford Aging Clinical Research Center, especially Ruth O'Hara.

Shelley Zulman was very helpful in getting us started on the manuscript, and particularly in helping us consider what it would take to make this material accessible to the full spectrum of audiences we hoped to reach. Without Donna Donovan's help in preparing and formatting the manuscript as well as her steady but always gracious and kind prodding, the production of this book would never have come in on anyone's schedule. We also want to thank Jane Nevins, who reviewed many sections of the manuscript and gave us very valuable advice. The last-minute reformatting of all the figures in the book was ably done by Brien Dilts, and we appreciate not only the skill and care with which this was done but also the speed with which it was accomplished.

At a more personal level, each of us owes a debt of gratitude to our families, who heard far more about "risk" than they probably ever wanted or expected to hear over much too long a time: Arthur and Stacey Kraemer, David Lowe, and Ellen Frank. And, finally, our inspirations: Jaylin and Lauren Lowe, granddaughters to the first author and daughters to the second; and Danielle, Adam, and Andrew Kupfer; Joshua, Noah, and Zachary Schneider; Lucy, Maddie, and Zoe Cosgrove; Yonatan and Nomi Strichman, all grandchildren of the last author. May these ideas lead to much better health to all of them in the near future!

Contents

Introduction

Why Did We Write This Book?

Cartoon by Jim Borgman. Reprinted with permission of King Features Syndicate.

Jim Borgman's cartoon sums up the confusion, maybe frustration, many of us feel when hearing of yet another report heralding new associations or new links between some characteristic, behavior, environment, or event and some outcome, usually one that we would all rather avoid.

Of course, scientists claim, many such reports are "hyped" by the media to be more interesting to the general consumer. Nevertheless, some of these reports are accurate accounts based on good research; others may be accurate but based on questionable research; and still others may be misleading

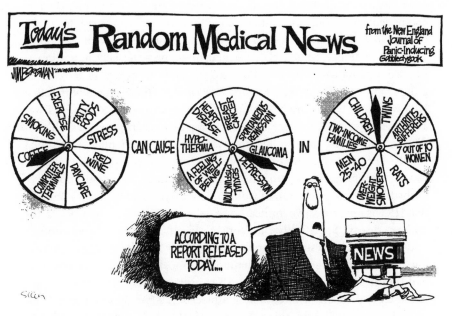

and misinterpreted statements based on either good or questionable research. The problem is: it's hard to tell what's credible and what's not, even if we go to the trouble of looking up the original reports in medical journals.

All of us can think of at least one occasion when we took such a report as a call to action, the basis of medical advice, or input into policy making, only to find a year or so later that other reports indicate that the action we took put us at risk for something else. Remember last year's efforts to increase carbohydrate consumption and reduce fats in our diet? Now should we reverse gears and minimize carbohydrates and include healthy fats? What will it be next year?

On a wider scale, consider what has happened to confuse and frighten millions of women about hormone replacement therapy (HRT). HRT is known to be therapeutic for hot flashes and other symptoms of menopause. Doctors and patients have long known that taking these hormones is a risk factor for certain types of cancer. However, HRT has been reported to prevent osteoporosis, cognitive decline, colorectal cancer, and, more controversially, heart disease. In 1985, contradictory back-to-back reports, both from reputable research groups, appeared in *The New England Journal of Medicine.* One reported that HRT was protective against heart disease,[1] and the other reported that HRT was a risk factor for heart disease.[2] How could top researchers generate such conflicting results, and how should clinicians and their patients react to such results? For some time thereafter, many doctors seemed to accept that HRT was, in fact, protective against heart disease and, on that assurance, prescribed HRT to a generation of women. Fifteen years later, studies indicate that HRT is *not* protective for heart disease and may actually be a risk factor for heart disease. Specifically, the Women's Health Initiative's large randomized clinical trial was stopped prematurely in July 2002 because women taking an estrogen-progestin combination (the most common form of HRT) had significantly more cases of breast cancer, strokes, heart attacks, and blood clots than did women taking a placebo.[3] After these reports, what should women currently taking this form of HRT do? Suddenly stop? Could a sudden stop lead to other problems?

An earlier example, from the 1970s, is perhaps more disturbing. At that time, evidence indicated that premature ventricular contractions (or PVCs—"extra" heartbeats that interrupt the normal heart rhythm[4]) were a major risk factor for heart attacks. The U.S. Food and Drug Administration approved drugs for prevention of heart attacks on the basis of evidence that they reduced PVCs.[5,6] In the years following, doctors wrote thousands of prescriptions for PVC-reducing drugs. Finally in the 1980s, the National Heart, Lung, and Blood Institute funded a randomized clinical trial comparing the effects of three such PVC-reducing drugs and a placebo on heart attacks. The study was closed down early because it became clear more deaths occurred among those taking the drug—a drug that was intended to reduce the risk of death, not increase it. It has been estimated that 10,000 premature deaths may be attributable to PVC-reducing drugs during the years prior to these studies.[5]

In recent years, a great deal of discussion has swirled around the value of mammography for routine screening for breast cancer in women,[7] and of prostate-specific antigen (PSA) for routine screening for prostate cancer in men.[8] In both cases, a false-positive result on the test can lead to invasive, costly, and sometimes even dangerous tests or treatments. In addition, some studies have suggested that these screening tests do not appreciably decrease the death rates for the relevant disorders. Is it possible that what these tests are detecting might often resolve without treatment or be just as treatable when detected later as when detected earlier?

When risk research regularly evolves from eye-catching headlines into catalysts for changing our lifestyles, prioritizing certain medical practices, or placing laws into practice, we must be concerned about inaccurate, overstated, mutually conflicting, or otherwise confusing information. Why are so many results confusing or conflicting when careful, dedicated medical researchers are doing their best to conduct accurate and informative research? In this book, we try to explain why studies often contradict each other and how researchers can reduce the ambiguity by changing the way they conduct research and communicate its results.

Medical risk research has three main components: risk estimation, risk evaluation, and risk management. In risk estimation, researchers attempt to identify particular characteristics linked to specific outcomes, with the goal of understanding the causes of diseases and disorders and developing interventions to prevent them. For example, a study that reports breast cancer is linked to antibiotics[9] is a risk estimation study. Risk evaluation and risk management also involve researchers as well as policy makers, physicians, consumer advocates, and all who seek to *evaluate* whether and *manage* how a research result should affect how they or others currently live their lives. For example, physicians acting as risk evaluators and managers might read the journal article describing the link between breast cancer and antibiotics and evaluate whether or not the result affects how and to whom they prescribe antibiotics.

We make a distinction here between these different components of risk research to acknowledge the importance of risk evaluation and risk management in medical decision making. In fact, from here on we will describe risk evaluation and risk management succinctly as "medical decision making." Nevertheless, our focus in this book is risk estimation. Risk estimation is based completely on scientific research, while medical decision making involves discourse, negotiation, and compromise among researchers as well as policy makers, physicians, and all who seek to use research results to improve their health and well-being.

Risk estimation that does not promote or progress to medical decisions is pointless. On the other hand, medical decisions not based on facts developed from risk estimation studies are perilous. Equally perilous are decisions based on risk estimation results that are faulty—and, to be blunt, much has been faulty. Even worse is risk estimation that is incomprehensible to decision makers and results that are too easily misunderstood or misinterpreted.

Much of what we will present aligns closely with the principles of "evidence-based medicine," an emerging trend in clinical practice today. Our focus, however, is on making sure that the "evidence" comes from well-designed and correctly interpreted risk estimation studies. Our goal is to prevent all involved in medical decision making—whether they are individual medical consumers, physicians, policy makers, or fellow researchers—from taking what could be damaging actions based on flawed or misrepresented risk estimation results. Specifically, for the medical consumer, we aim to provide the tools to recognize good research and understand if it is important and to whom it is important. In addition, for the medical professional and researcher, we recommend new techniques and conceptualizations of the research process with the goal of ultimately increasing the value of the risk estimation conducted currently and in the future.

Although much of risk estimation falls in the area of medical research called epidemiology, this is not a basic epidemiology textbook, not least because epidemiologists may disagree with some of what we say. Epidemiology is defined in *A Dictionary of Epidemiology* as "the study of the distribution and determinants of health-related states or events in specified populations, and the application of this study to control of health problems."[10(p55)] Although this definition coincides closely with how we have described risk estimation, not all of epidemiology is risk estimation, and not all risk estimation is done by epidemiologists. Risk estimation involves clinical researchers in all fields of medicine, as well as psychologists, sociologists, and others. Many of the terms we precisely define for the purpose of risk estimation are used more loosely in the epidemiology literature. Many of the methods we criticize as a basis for medical decisions are acceptable to epidemiologists using them for other purposes. At the same time, we do not use or advocate some of the terms and methods basic to epidemiology.

We have divided this book into four parts. Part I provides the basic principles required for understanding and correctly communicating the results of risk estimation (Chapters 1–5). We emphasize how simple miscommunication about what a risk factor is, how important a risk factor is, and how a risk factor can be used is often the source of current confusion and sometimes leads to possibly harmful actions not actually supported by the research results. Part I includes sometimes amusing and sometimes aggravating examples, most drawn from the public media, of how research is correctly and incorrectly conducted, interpreted, and presented. We hope these chapters will be interesting and thought provoking but, most important, we hope they will provide an introductory guide for determining what to believe and what not to believe about risk factors.

Part II (Chapters 6–8) expands on many of the basic principles from Part I concerning research design. We enlarge our argument from the value of understanding precisely what a risk factor is and what appropriate uses a risk factor might serve to how to recognize good research, and therefore which results to trust and which to doubt. We argue that researchers can do a better job designing studies, and consumers should demand that they do better. We make clear why certain methods can make studies more trustworthy—and that nonexperts can discern whether such methods underlie any published study. Although here we draw examples from the research literature, rather than the public media, Part II is no more technical than Part I. Our goal for Part II is to provide the tools for any reader to recognize the "danger signs" of bad research and to be able to decipher whether and in what way a particular research result is relevant.

Part III (Chapters 9–11) is directed more specifically to a reader who will be involved in conducting research, analyzing research results, and communicating such results. Although someone who has taken one or more courses in research methods or statistical analysis will find the going easier, we don't assume extensive statistical training and have done all we can to introduce the technical topics with ample explanation and references to the technical literature for further study. Chapters 9–11 discuss methodological approaches to risk estimation aimed at producing interpretable and reproducible results. We think everyone will find this information enlightening, but the nonresearcher does not need to understand this material perfectly to read Part IV or to achieve the goals of this book.

Part IV (Chapters 12–14) is our own call to action. We believe changes in how medical researchers conduct and communicate their research, as well as how others interpret and describe it, will improve future risk research and avoid the dangerous reversals we have witnessed too many times in recent years.

Our overall goal for this book is to make every reader a smart skeptic and thereby encourage a shift in the course of future risk research. Poor-quality risk estimation will persist until all of us understand the process better and until we make it clear that we are no longer willing to see taxpayer or philanthropic money spent on unnecessary or flawed research. We also hope that the ideas and approaches described in this book will reduce the amount of erroneous advice based on unsubstantiated claims and prevent decision makers from enacting policy or individuals taking drastic action without careful consideration of the adequacy of research methods and interpretation. The consequences of poor risk research cannot be ignored when the ultimate cost may be the shortened duration and diminished quality of human life.

I

The Basics of Risk

1

What Is Risk?

A census taker is a man who goes from house to house increasing the population.

He wanted an heir to inherit his power, but since Josephine was a baroness, she couldn't bear children.

Under the Constitution the people enjoyed the right to keep bare arms.

A scout obeys all to whom obedience is due and respects all duly constipated authorities.

Acrimony, sometimes called holy, is another name for marriage.

A monologue is a conversation between two people, such as husband and wife.

It is a well-known fact that a deceased body harms the mind.

It's hard not to laugh when children misuse words and say something different from what they intended. Even when adults make such mistakes in casual conversation, the results can be funny. However, when adults miscommunicate in noncasual conversations, and (particularly for our purposes) when such miscommunication occurs in scientific or policy applications, the results may be catastrophic. For example, recall the 1999 multimillion-dollar debacle that resulted in the loss of a space probe to Mars when the spacecraft designers and builders unwittingly communicated in different measurement units.[1]

Risk research is one of the many contexts where clear and correct communication is vital. Misunderstandings or miscommunications in risk research can affect everyone—from the risk researchers themselves to the health care providers, to the ultimate "consumers" of risk research—anyone seeking guidance with respect to his or her health. For example, consider the newspaper headline in Example 1.1.

EXAMPLE 1.1

In a study described in an article titled "Study Links Sleeping to Attention Problems,"[2] researchers questioned parents about their children's sleep habits, distractibility, forgetfulness, and fidgeting. Researchers found that kids who snored were more likely to also exhibit symptoms of hyperactivity.

How should we react to a report such as the one described in Example 1.1? What exactly does "links" mean? Would you be tempted to describe snoring as a risk factor for hyperactivity or hyperactivity as a risk factor for snoring? Would you be surprised to hear speculation about whether snoring *causes* hyperactivity or hyperactivity *causes* snoring? Should we have our own hyperactive child evaluated for sleep disturbances or our child who snores evaluated for hyperactivity?

The words researchers choose to describe such results and the words we use to think about them have a direct impact on how we might respond. These words are critical to considerations of our own health, as well as critical to guiding future research. Even though no words were imprecisely used in the original description describing the "link" between sleep and attention problems, often the words we, reporters, or other researchers may use—words such as "risk factor" and even "cause"—are casually chosen, changing the interpretation of the original report.

In Chapters 1–3, we take the first steps toward helping readers become smart skeptics by defining the basic terms. In this chapter, we begin with the term "risk" and build upon that definition in later chapters to define "risk factor," "causal risk factor," and others. Although all of us are probably familiar with terms such as "risk," "risk factor," and "cause," these terms in particular have been inconsistently and imprecisely used to the detriment of scientific advancement.[3] We strive to provide one consistent set of definitions, but to do so, we will at times present definitions that are not exactly the same as the definitions of the same terms used in other fields. In addition, we will also introduce some terms (e.g., "correlate" and "proxy risk factor") that may be different than the typical terms used by some researchers. Nevertheless, in order to provide a consistent framework and language throughout this book, we must stick to one term with one definition in hopes that others will follow suit. In presenting these definitions, we stress that clear and precise communication is necessary to recognize when a result has been inappropriately interpreted and to avoid making inappropriate interpretations ourselves.

What Is Risk?

In casual conversation, the word "risk" is used in different contexts to mean different things. Even when we limit ourselves to only those contexts that involve health, "risk" can refer to the chance of an outcome (as in "the risk of death while skydiving"), or it can refer to the outcome itself (as in "a risk of skydiving is death"). Semantically, both these uses (and others) are correct. However, to achieve clarity and consistency in the basic terms of risk research, we need to stick to one precise definition of risk.

Risk: The probability of an outcome within a population.[3]

In our definition of risk, a "population" is a group of people with particular common characteristics (e.g., women, Americans, children under the age of five). An "outcome" is a health-related event or condition (e.g., whether or not a person has cancer, diabetes, or depression). Examples of risk according to this definition include "the risk of breast cancer among women over age 50," "the risk of autism among preschool-aged children," and "the risk of a heart attack within one year among men younger than 45 years." As short and simple as this definition of risk is, it has three critical and distinct implications, each discussed in turn below:

1. Risk is a *probability.*
2. Researchers measure risk within a well-specified *population.*
3. Researchers measure risk for a precisely specified *outcome.*

Risk Is a Probability

The probability of an outcome in a population conveys how likely a person in that population will have the outcome. Researchers *estimate* this probability by selecting a specific number of people from the population of interest ("study participants") and calculating the percentage of the study participants who have the outcome. Consequently, a risk is some number between 0% and 100% (or a fraction between 0 and 1) where the outcome (for our purposes) is health-related—contracting a disease or a disorder, recovering from a disease, remission, death, and so forth.

Notice how we have included desirable outcomes (recovery and remission) as well as undesirable outcomes (contracting a disease or disorder, death) in our list of health-related outcomes for risk estimation. Since the goal of risk estimation is to identify what causes certain diseases or disorders, risk researchers are as interested to discover what "goes right" as what "goes wrong." We can as correctly say "the risk of contracting breast cancer" as we can say "the risk of *not* contracting breast cancer." Nevertheless, we cannot avoid the implied negative connotations of the word "risk." For this reason, we will tend to use additional clarifying words when talking about the risk of desirable outcomes.

Also notice how these desirable or undesirable outcomes either occur or not—an individual has a disease or not, recovers or still has the disease, lives or dies. For researchers to calculate the risk of an outcome, the outcome must be binary. Although other important medical research involve predicting nonbinary outcomes (e.g., cholesterol level, HIV viral load, the number of weeks until remission from cancer, etc.), the goals of such research differ from the goals of risk estimation in predicting who will and who will not have a particular outcome.

Finally, if risk is a probability, what does it mean to speak about "my risk" or "your risk" for a particular outcome? How does a researcher figure out "your risk"? Everyone has an individual probability at any point in time to, for example, have a heart attack in the next five years. This individual probability depends on all the genetic, biological, environmental, and lifestyle influences we have accumulated to date. Unfortunately, researchers cannot measure the probability for an individual. They can only study a group with characteristics similar to an individual and count how many people in that group had the outcome of interest. Thus, "your risk" is estimated by studying a group of people similar to you. The more similar the study group is to you, the closer that estimated risk comes to your unknown individual probability.

For example, suppose your cholesterol levels have always been considered "normal." However, you now hear from your doctor that your cholesterol profile measured last week has exceeded some threshold, indicating that you are now considered at high risk for a heart attack within five years. Did your risk change? Are you suddenly more likely to have a heart attack than you were two weeks ago before you had your blood drawn?

The probability you actually will have a heart attack has probably not changed much in the last two weeks. Nevertheless, today when your doctor discovered you have high cholesterol, your doctor's *estimate* of your risk of a heart attack within the next five years did change. That is, your doctor now recognizes that you are more likely than before to have a heart attack in the next five years because the risk among people *like you* is higher.

Your risk is described by the proportion of people like you who experienced a particular outcome, as shown in risk studies. Your risk is considered high or low if the population of people like you is more or less likely to experience the outcome than a reference population, typically the general population. For example, a 15% risk of death in the next five years for a 20-year-old might be considered high because among all 20-year-olds many fewer than 15% will die in the next five years. However, a 15% risk of death in the next five years for a 90-year-old might be considered low because among all 90-year-olds, more than 15% will probably die before their 95th birthday. In other words, people use "high risk" or "low risk" to mean higher or lower risk than some reference population.

Thus, to understand risk we must carefully define what population we are considering, bringing us to the second important implication of our definition of risk, that researchers measure risk within a well-specified population.

Researchers Measure Risk within a Well-Specified Population

When researchers measure the risk of death in the next five years, they will find that that risk is much higher for 90-year-olds than for 20-year-olds. Similarly, the risk of lung cancer among smokers is not the same as the risk of lung cancer in the general population, and the risk of lung cancer among men is not the same as the risk of lung cancer among women. The results from a risk estimation study using one population do not necessarily apply to another, different population. Consider Examples 1.2 and 1.3.

EXAMPLE 1.2

Early research estimating the risk of breast cancer among women with mutations in certain genes (specifically, the *BRCA1* and *BRCA2* genes) suggested that women with these mutations had a lifetime risk of breast cancer of 80% or more. This frightening statistic must have convinced some women with these mutations to consider having their breasts removed in hopes of preventing breast cancer. Now, however, experts believe these risks may have been exaggerated. Many of the early studies sampled women whose sisters, mothers, and grandmothers had breast cancer. For women with *both* the mutation *and* the family history, the risk may indeed be that high. However, for those with only the mutation—a different and much larger population—drastic and irreversible decisions may have resulted from this misinformation.[4]

EXAMPLE 1.3

The American Heart Association published the following statistics for men and for women (from the Framingham Heart Study, National Heart, Lung, and Blood Institute):[5]

- The risk of death within a year of a first recognized heart attack is 38% for women and 25% for men.
- The risk of another heart attack within six years of a recognized heart attack is 35% for women and 18% for men.
- The risk of being disabled with heart failure within six years of a recognized heart attack is 46% for women and 22% for men.

Note how the risk estimates in Example 1.3 are very different for men than for women. Likewise, how this risk changes as we age is different for men than for women. Research results from one population may simply be different in another population.

Years ago, researchers tended to focus their research efforts on limited populations (e.g., studying heart disease in men only) and assumed the results applied to other populations. Now differences in populations are widely recognized, and the National Institutes of Health stresses the necessity of including women, minorities, and children in research. Nevertheless, subtle but possibly significant differences in populations can also lead to very different results, as mentioned in Example 1.2 concerning the risk of breast cancer among women with and without a family history of the disease. Likewise, studies of well-educated people with good access to medical care (e.g., doctors or nurses) may not apply to socioeconomically disadvantaged individuals. Consider Example 1.4, another current example in which the result of a study of a very specific population has been extended by many to other, possibly very different, populations.

EXAMPLE 1.4

A pharmaceutical company sponsored a study to show that two different statins (drugs prescribed to lower cholesterol) were equivalent. However, researchers were surprised to discover these two drugs were *not* equivalent. Study participants taking the intense statin therapy had a much lower LDL level (the "bad" cholesterol) and a lower rate of heart attacks, heart surgeries and other procedures, and death than did those taking the moderate statin therapy.[6] In all the excitement following the result, when doctors were quoted as saying, "We have in our hands the power to reduce the risk of heart disease by a lot," and "Everyone needs to shift up one level in their intensity of cholesterol treatment,"[7] rarely did the newspaper articles describing the result emphasize that the study population consisted of 4,162 hospitalized patients who had just suffered either a heart attack or sudden acute chest pain. Surely this population is different than those of us with slightly elevated LDL cholesterol who have never been hospitalized and have no other indication of heart disease. Nevertheless, some have interpreted the result to mean intense statin therapy is better, in general.

Perhaps intense statin therapy is better in preventing heart-related events, even given the additional side effects of taking the more intensive therapy, but certainly the study described in Example 1.4 does not support that conclusion for anyone except those already experiencing serious heart-related events.

The onus is on the researchers to communicate *exactly* what population they studied and to take care not to overgeneralize results beyond the limits of that population. The onus is on the health care provider, the policy maker, and the consumer to evaluate that information carefully and decide whether the results are pertinent to their needs.

Researchers Measure Risk for a Precisely Specified Outcome

Besides checking the population studied, anyone considering the relevance of a particular study needs to check how researchers defined the outcome. That is, how did the researchers determine whether or not a study participant had, for example, diabetes? Just as a risk estimate within two different populations may vary considerably, risk estimates for differently defined outcomes concerning the same health issue can also vary.

Outcomes for the same health issue can differ in what diagnostic criteria the researchers used to determine whether or not the study participant had the outcome of interest. For many outcomes, this is simple: Is the participant alive or dead? Others may not be so simple: Is the participant "severely depressed"? (Doctors can use different criteria to diagnose and describe depression, and different doctors might have different diagnoses.) Or does the participant have "high cholesterol"? (The researcher would have to define high cholesterol—e.g., total cholesterol greater than 200 mg/dl or LDL cholesterol greater than 150 mg/dl.)

Outcomes for the same health issue can also differ in more subtle, but important, ways. For example, when doctors started using the prostate-specific antigen (PSA) test to screen for prostate cancer, many more men were diagnosed early with prostate cancers. However, more diagnoses of prostate cancer have not necessarily translated into a significantly lower death rate from prostate cancer.[8] Thus, if researchers use the diagnosis of prostate cancer as an outcome when studying the value of the PSA test, they may get a different answer than if they define the outcome as death from prostate cancer. The same may be true when researchers study the value of mammography in detecting breast cancer. Since the introduction of mammography, the number of breast cancer diagnoses has risen, suggesting more cancers are being detected with the screening test. However, the number of cancers that had spread to other organs—that is, the worst of the cases—has not changed dramatically since mammography was introduced, suggesting that use of mammography has not decreased the number of cancers most likely to result in death.[9] Thus, when researchers study the value of these cancer screening tests, they have to carefully consider what is the important outcome—the diagnosis of cancer or death from cancer?

Even when researchers define the exact same outcome, they may specify a different time period over which the outcome can occur. For example, the risk of death for a 20-year-old is trivially identical to the risk of death for a 90-year-old, because all 20-year-olds and all 90-year-olds must eventually experience death. However, their risks differ immensely if we specify when that death occurs, such as within the next five years. Typically, we will hear risk estimates such as "the risk of a heart attack within five years," "the risk of colon cancer within ten years," and so forth.

Finally, even when researchers select the same criteria and time period to determine whether or not a participant has an outcome, researchers can make one other important and sometimes confusing distinction in determining whether or not a participant is considered to have the outcome. Researchers can consider a study participant as having the outcome if the *onset* of the outcome occurs during the specified time period. Alternatively, researchers can consider a study participant as having the outcome if he or she experiences the outcome during the time period *regardless of when the onset occurred.* The distinction between these two ways of determining whether a participant is counted as having the outcome makes the most difference when the outcome of interest occurs in episodes. Episodic outcomes are those in which a person after onset of conditions such as asthma, psoriasis, depression, and schizophrenia is sometimes symptomatic and sometimes not. For example, the risk for a woman of ever experiencing depression within a lifetime might be 20%. In a specific one-year period, 6% or 7% of women might experience depression. In that same one-year period, 3–4% of women might have onset of depression. All three of these estimates are risk estimates of outcomes concerning depression using the same criteria to diagnose depression, but their values and interpretations may be very different. The first risk estimate is referred to as a "lifetime prevalence," the second a "prevalence," and the third an "incidence."

An "incidence" is the risk of an outcome in which *onset* of the disease occurs within a specified period of time (think of new cases coming "in"). A "prevalence" is the risk of an outcome in which a person experiences the outcome within the specified period of time—*regardless of when the onset occurred* (think of "prevalent," i.e., existing). So, for example, short-lived diseases, such as the flu, have a high annual incidence (many people will get the flu during a one-year period) but a low prevalence during any month—particularly during a summer month. Chronic diseases, such as diabetes, have a low yearly incidence (many who have the disorder in a particular year would have been diagnosed earlier) but a high yearly prevalence (including both the incident cases and those diagnosed earlier).[10] Figure 1.1 illustrates the differences between incidence and prevalence by depicting hypothetical time courses of a disease for six people over a five-year period.

Researchers use both incidence and prevalence validly in risk research. Sometimes one is more appropriate; at other times, the other is more appro-

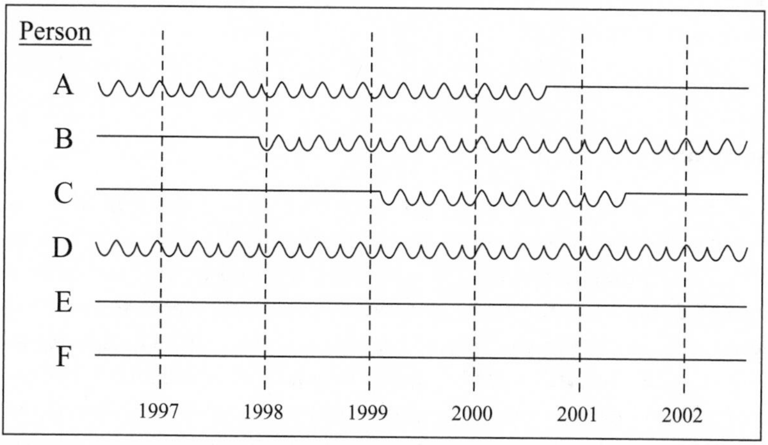

Figure 1.1. An illustration of the difference between incidence and prevalence. For a hypothetical five-year period, curved lines represent times when a person has the disease; straight lines represent times when a person does not have the disease. Person A had onset prior to the time period and recovered during the time period. Person B had onset during the time period and recovered after the time period. Person C has both onset and recovery within the time period. Person D had onset prior to the time period and never recovered during the time period. Persons E and F never had the disease during the time period. Persons B and C had onset of the disease during the time period; the incidence is 2/6 = 33%. Persons A, B, C, and D experienced the disease during the time period; the prevalence is 4/6 = 66%.

priate. However, a "lifetime prevalence" is an even trickier concept. For example, most of us have probably heard the frightening statistic that one in eight or nine women will be diagnosed with breast cancer in her lifetime.[11] The implied interpretation of this "lifetime prevalence" is that of all women born in, say, 1970, one out of eight of them will be diagnosed with breast cancer before her death or at autopsy.

Researchers use many different methods for estimating lifetime prevalence. One common way often seen in the psychiatric epidemiology literature is to calculate the proportion of people who answer "yes" to the question "Have you ever had this outcome?" The answer to this question depends on the ages of the selected participants. Someone who answers "no" at age 20 may answer "yes" at age 40. The "lifetime prevalence" tends to be higher the older the age distribution in a particular study and may differ greatly from one study to another. Consequently, lifetime prevalence is very difficult to accurately estimate or interpret.

Thus, just as we urge the necessity to check what population researchers studied, anyone considering a result needs to check how researchers defined the outcome, while researchers must carefully communicate how they defined that outcome. Not all outcomes relating to the same disorder or disease are equal.

Conclusion and Summary

When it comes to comprehending the results of risk estimation, the words used either by the original researcher or by anyone describing the result are critical for guiding how we think about and respond to the result. For this reason, we stress—to the researcher, the reporter, and everyone considering a result—the importance of correctly using the terms central to risk research.

In this chapter, we focused on the term that is the foundation for all other terms: *risk*. We defined risk as the probability of an outcome within a population, stressing the importance of carefully scrutinizing who the people in the study were (the population) and exactly how the outcome is defined. If the people studied are not similar to the person or people for whom you are seeking a risk estimate or if the outcome is one you are interested in but is defined in a way not relevant to your needs, then the result also may not be relevant.

Rarely, however, are we interested in a simple risk estimate for a population. Knowing that the risk is 17% or 23% does not typically affect medical decision making unless we also know how to lower that risk (for undesirable outcomes) or raise that risk (for desirable outcomes). What we really care about are the characteristics, environments, and behaviors—more generically put, the "factors"—that put us at higher or lower risk and ideally whether and how we can change those factors to change our risk. That is, we care about risk as a means to discover risk factors, perhaps causes, and eventually understand how certain outcomes can be prevented or promoted. Thus, our purpose for carefully defining risk is to build upon that definition to define risk factors and the different types of risk factors, including causal risk factors.

- Clear and precise communication is essential to risk research. Although all of us are familiar with the terms "risk," "risk factor," and "cause," sometimes these terms are casually interchanged, possibly misguiding how we think about or act upon new risk research results.
- Risk is the probability of an outcome within a population.
- For risk estimation, the outcome is binary (for each study participant, the outcome of interest either occurs or does not occur) and may be desirable (e.g., remission, recovery from disease) or undesirable (e.g., disease or death).
- Researchers measure risk within a well-specified population. Researchers must clearly communicate what this population is. Individuals wanting to use the findings must carefully check that this population is similar to the one to which they wish to apply the findings. An estimated risk of an outcome in one population (e.g., the risk of heart disease among American men 40–50 years of age) may not apply in another population (e.g., the risk of heart disease among American women 40–50 years of age or American men 60–70 years of age).
- Researchers measure risk for a precisely specified outcome. Risk estimates of outcomes concerning the same health issue, but defined differently, may be quite different. Researchers must specify the diagnostic criteria used to determine whether a study participant has the outcome or not. Researchers must specify a time period (e.g., death in five years). Finally, they must specify whether they consider a participant as having the outcome if onset of the outcome occurs during the time period of interest (incidence) or whether the study participant simply experiences the outcome at some point during the time period (prevalence).
- "Lifetime prevalence" is sometimes a misleading estimate of risk. We advise care in interpreting lifetime prevalence.

2

What Is a Risk Factor?

"Breast Is Best for Better Brains"

"Breast Milk Found to Cut Leukemia Risk"

"Adventurous Toddlers Score Higher in IQ Study"

"Working Moms' Kids Less Ready for School"

"TV May 'Rewire' Children's Brains"

Should we urge all mothers to stay home, breast-feed their infants, and encourage their toddlers to be adventurous while not allowing them to watch television? Each of these newspaper headlines[1–5] describes how certain characteristics, behaviors, environments, or events (or more succinctly put, certain "factors") are "associated with," are "linked to," or somehow are related to specific outcomes. Do these relationships mean these factors are risk factors? If they are, how should we consider and react to them? If they are not, what are they?

In this chapter, we answer these questions by defining more of the terms central to risk research. Specifically, we will clarify what is a risk factor and, possibly more important, what is not a risk factor.

What Does It Mean for a Factor to Be "Linked" to an Outcome?

Researchers will report a factor is "linked" to an outcome to indicate that they have demonstrated that certain values of the factor are more often seen among those having the outcome (or vice versa). For example, we can say gender is linked to color blindness, meaning that the risk of being color-blind is different for males than for females. If you were asked to guess the gender of a color-blind person, and you knew that the risk of color blindness is higher for males than for females, you would be right more often than not if you were to guess "male."

Other words that are used interchangeably with "link" are "relationship," "association," and a "correlation" between a factor and an outcome. How researchers demonstrate a link, relationship, association, and correlation is the subject of Chapter 4. For our purposes here, however, what is important is that a relationship or an association exists between a factor and an outcome when knowing whether or not a person has the outcome gives you information about his or her value for the factor (e.g., whether the person is male or female, or the person's cholesterol level) or, alternatively, when knowing that person's value of the factor gives you information about whether or not he or she has the outcome.

Correlate: A factor that is shown to be associated with an outcome within a population.

We describe a factor that is associated with an outcome as a "correlate." Notice that our definition of correlate specifically describes a correlate with reference to a population. Just as estimates of risks may vary from population to population, an association within one population may be different from that in another population, as in Example 2.1.

EXAMPLE 2.1

Married teenage girls are more likely to commit suicide than are unmarried teenage girls. However, married adult women are less likely to commit suicide than are unmarried adult women.[6–9]

Although whether or not a person is married is a correlate of the outcome (suicide) both among teenage girls and among adult women, the relationship between marriage and suicide described in Example 2.1 is opposite in these two different populations. That is, among teenage girls, marriage is associated with a *higher* risk of suicide, while among adult women, marriage is associated with a *lower* risk of suicide. Since marriage and suicide are associated within two different populations, by our definition, marriage is a correlate of suicide in each of these populations. But is marriage, then, a risk factor for suicide within each of these two populations?

What Is a Risk Factor?

> *Risk factor: A correlate that* is shown to precede *the outcome.*[10]

The marriage for either the teenage girl or the adult woman preceded her death, so by our definition, marriage is a risk factor for suicide among both teenage girls and adult women. Just as risk is not necessarily the probability of an *undesirable* outcome, a risk factor does not have to predict an *undesirable* outcome. Although the term "risk factor" describes any factor that can distinguish those of "high risk" from those of "low risk" of an outcome—whether desirable or undesirable—to avoid confusion, we will usually describe a factor that predicts a welcome outcome as a "protective factor." Specifically, we will say, "Marriage is a protective factor against suicide among adult women" in contrast to, "Marriage is a risk factor for suicide among teenage girls."

That key distinction between a correlate and a risk factor, the *temporal precedence* of the factor, relates to what is perhaps the most common mistake in risk research: calling a factor, shown only to be a correlate, a risk factor. Researchers want to discover risk factors in order to *predict* who is at highest risk for an outcome and, ideally, to intervene *before* the outcome occurs. For example, researchers are looking for risk factors to predict when a woman might become infertile.[11] Since more and more women today are delaying childbearing, researchers one day hope to be able to test a young woman's future fertility so that she can make informed choices. Of course, women will not benefit from researchers' efforts unless they can predict infertility *before* infertility occurs. Since the goal of risk research is to prevent undesirable or promote desirable outcomes, a risk factor must precede the outcome in order to offer any possibility of predicting and then preventing or promoting the outcome.

Correlates, on the other hand, may be risk factors, but they also may be symptoms of the outcome that has already occurred or may be the consequences of that outcome. For example, the fever, muscle aches, and congestion that accompany the flu are not risk factors for the flu but symptoms of the flu. The abdominal scar that is left after an appendectomy is not a risk factor for an inflamed appendix but a consequence of an inflamed appendix. Only when we know that a correlate existed prior to the outcome do we call it a risk factor for that outcome (see Figure 2.1). *All risk factors are correlates, but not all correlates are risk factors.*

Establishing precedence is often not an easy task. Researchers have no problem showing that a correlate precedes an outcome when the outcome is

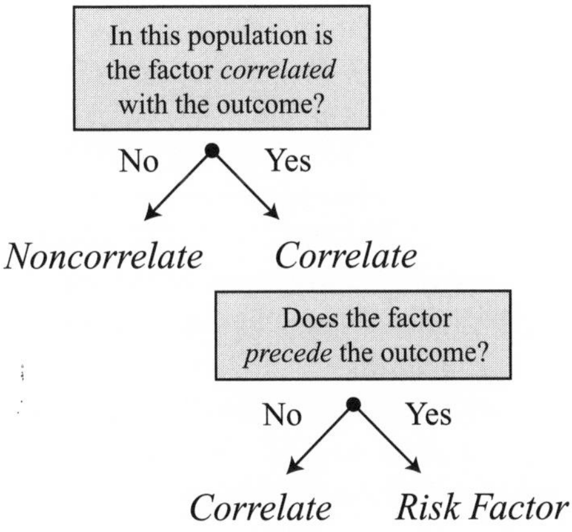

Figure 2.1. A flowchart distinguishing correlates from risk factors.

death. However, if instead we consider an outcome such as "having suicidal thoughts," then establishing precedence is much more challenging. Researchers often conduct studies at one point in time ("cross-sectional studies"), with both the factors and outcomes being measured simultaneously. Such studies are generally easy and less costly to do. For example, researchers may ask teenagers "Are you married?" and, at the same time, ask "Have you ever had suicidal thoughts?" If researchers do discover a relationship between the study participants' answers to these two questions, they can only describe marriage as a correlate for the suicidal thoughts among teenagers, because the researchers did not show whether a teenager's suicidal thoughts came before or after the marriage.

Consider Example 2.2 (which we've also discussed in Chapter 1), an example that comes from a cross-sectional study.

EXAMPLE 2.2

In a study described in an article titled "Study Links Sleeping to Attention Problems,"[12] researchers questioned parents about their children's sleep habits, distractibility, forgetfulness, and fidgeting. Researchers found that kids who snored were more likely to also exhibit symptoms of hyperactivity.

In Example 2.2, researchers compared parents' reports of hyperactivity traits to reports of sleep habits. Can we conclude that the sleep disturbances lead to hyperactivity? Is it possible that instead, hyperactivity fosters sleep problems? Both explanations are plausible, but then which is the risk factor and which is the outcome? Since researchers asked about sleep habits and hyperactivity simultaneously, there is no way to know which comes first. Until we know the directionality of the association, if any, further research could be misled, and practitioners might be misled to "treat" the wrong symptoms and potentially cause more confusion and harm.

Example 2.2 also brings up another issue that warrants some attention. Consider two additional explanations for the association between children's sleep habits and hyperactivity. Perhaps the stress induced by the child's hyperactivity disturbs the parents' sleep, making the parents more aware of what is happening with the child during the night, causing them to over-report sleep problems. Alternatively, perhaps the parents are so exhausted from attending to their child's sleep disturbances that they report more negatively on their child's daytime behavior, creating a misclassification of the child as hyperactive. In short, the fact that researchers for this study used parental reports to measure both the factor and the outcome raises concerns about the interpretation of the results. Reports of snoring and behavioral problems may be linked only because the same person (the parent) reported on both. When researchers collect retrospective self-reports after the outcome may have occurred, the fact that the outcome did or did not occur does sometimes change how people perceive, recall, and describe events prior to the outcome.

Retrospective self-report can be valuable if collected *before* the outcome of interest. That is, instead of conducting a cross-sectional study, researchers can conduct a "longitudinal study" and follow study participants, none of whom had the outcome at the start of the study, for a period of time to see if the outcome occurs. If researchers ask the study participants to provide a self-report before the outcome of interest occurs, then that self-report can be a risk factor for the outcome. Even though self-reports are not always reliable accounts of what really happened, the report itself can be a risk factor even if it is an inaccurate account of past events. For example, an adult's retrospective report of childhood sexual abuse may be a risk factor for subsequent onset of depression, even if the abuse never occurred. That is, the perception or interpretation of past experiences as abusive may itself be a risk factor for subsequent onset of depression.[10] In general, retrospective self-reports must be interpreted with care.

Before researchers demonstrate association and precedence of a factor, we should not use words such as correlate or risk factor. We might reasonably refer to factors *hypothesized* to be risk factors as "potential risk factors." Assumptions and hypotheses can be and, unfortunately, have at times been wrong.

Are All Risk Factors Equal?

We use risk factors to predict whether or not an individual will, at a later date, have an outcome ideally so we can do something to prevent or delay its onset (or promote a desirable outcome). Thus, risk factors not only identify who will have the outcome but may also provide a basis for an intervention to prevent or promote that outcome. For example, doctors may use high cholesterol level or high blood pressure to predict who might be at greater risk for cardiovascular diseases. Part of the intervention doctors might provide for those patients considered high risk may involve medications to reduce cholesterol and/or blood pressure. In this case, the risk factors, blood pressure and cholesterol level, both identify those who are high risk and suggest an intervention for those who are high risk. However, changing risk factors does not necessarily change the risk of the outcome. Moreover, while any risk factor can help identify those at higher risk of an outcome, not all suggest a basis for an intervention. For example, gender is a risk factor that can help identify who is high risk for many outcomes, such as early heart disease and depression, but gender is not a risk factor that can be changed to prevent or promote an outcome. In Chapter 3, we describe the different types of risk factors and how each can (and cannot) be used.

Risk factors are not all equal in terms of what functions they might serve, but they are also not all equal in terms of their ability to predict an outcome. When researchers demonstrate a relationship between a risk factor and an outcome, they usually demonstrate that people with the risk factor have a "statistically significant" higher (or lower) risk of the outcome. What really matters, however, is not statistical significance, but how much higher is that risk in the "high risk" population than in the "low risk" population. Such clinical or policy significance is sometimes overlooked in the presentation of a new risk factor. Researchers, reporters, physicians, and medical consumers can get excited that a new interesting link has been discovered (e.g., "Exercise Aids Cancer Recovery, Study Says"[13]), and forget to ask, "How much difference does it make?" We devote Chapter 4 to statistical significance and how much a risk factor matters, but for now, our message is that some risk factors are more useful than others both in terms of their function and in terms of how well they predict an outcome.

Conclusion and Summary

The definition of "risk factor" requires that researchers demonstrate the factor precedes the outcome. When researchers cannot establish precedence—typically because they measured the correlate and outcome simultaneously—there is a "chicken-and-egg" problem of figuring out which is the risk factor and which is the outcome.

Even when a correlate is correctly described as such, if other researchers, doctors, and medical consumers interpret the correlate as a risk factor (and particularly if they interpret it as a "cause"), they may consider taking action on the basis of misleading information. As a result, research dollars may be wasted because researchers are looking at the wrong outcome or health might be jeopardized if individuals take action to change a correlate that ultimately has no effect on preventing the outcome.

However, taking action to change a bona fide risk factor also may have no effect on preventing the outcome. While all risk factors identify people who are high risk for the outcome, some risk factors also can form the bases of interventions intended to change that risk of the outcome. In this chapter, we concentrated on simply defining what is and is not a risk factor. In Chapter 3 we further that discussion to define the different types and the different uses of risk factors.

- A factor is linked (or equivalently, is associated/correlated/has a relationship) with an outcome when researchers demonstrate some relationship such that certain values of the factor are more often seen with either having or not having the outcome (e.g., gender is associated with color blindness since many more men are color-blind than are women).
- A correlate is a factor that is shown to be associated with an outcome within a population.
- A risk factor is a correlate that is shown to precede an outcome.
- All risk factors are correlates but not all correlates are risk factors.
- The distinction between a correlate and a risk factor is important because only what happens before an outcome gives clues as to possible causes of the outcome. In addition, only before the outcome occurs can you hope to intervene and prevent (or promote) the outcome.
- A risk factor for a welcome outcome is still a risk factor but, for clarity, may be referred to as a "protective factor."
- Not all risk factors are equal. Some risk factors can only identify who is at high risk of an outcome (e.g., gender). Other risk factors can both identify who is at high risk and serve as the basis of an intervention to prevent or promote that outcome. Not only are risk factors not equal in terms of their function, but some are more accurate than others in predicting an outcome (more "potent"). A risk factor's potency is an important consideration when evaluating whether or not a risk factor matters.

3

Are All Risk Factors Equal?

Types of Risk Factors

> *The Bell Curve,* with its claims and supposed documentation that race and class differences are largely caused by genetic factors and are therefore essentially immutable, contains no new arguments and presents no compelling data to support its anachronistic social Darwinism, so I can only conclude that its success in winning attention must reflect the depressing temper of our time—a historical moment of unprecedented ungenerosity, when a mood for slashing social programs can be powerfully abetted by an argument that beneficiaries cannot be helped, owing to inborn cognitive limits expressed as low IQ scores.
>
> —Stephen J. Gould's comment on the 1994 national best-seller *The Bell Curve*

Race and ethnicity are well-documented risk factors for low IQ and other associated outcomes such as poor school performance and low socioeconomic level. Many research studies have demonstrated the link between race and ethnicity and low IQ with no major outcry from scientists. Why, then, such outcry against *The Bell Curve,* as illustrated by Gould's comment?[1(p11)] We cannot change risk factors such as race, but does that mean that nothing can be done to prevent low IQ as suggested by *The Bell Curve*? Moreover, risk factors often associated with race, such as poor health care and poor schooling, are changeable, but can we be sure that changing them will reduce the likelihood of low IQ?

Whether a risk factor can change and whether changing it makes a difference to the outcome are the main criteria distinguishing the different types of risk factors. Recognizing these different types is the key to understanding what we *can* and *cannot* do with risk factors.

What Can We Do with a Risk Factor That Cannot Change?

In risk estimation, researchers are looking for things we *can* do to prevent or promote an outcome—take a drug, go on a diet, exercise, stop smoking, and so on. However, if a risk factor cannot change, we cannot hope that changing it might prevent or promote an outcome. We describe such an unchangeable risk factor as a "fixed marker."

> *Fixed marker: A risk factor that cannot change or be changed.*

Examples of potential fixed markers include gender, race/ethnicity, year of birth, genotype, eye color, skin color, and whether or not someone was born prematurely. For example, two fixed markers for being HIV positive are having hemophilia and being born in Africa. Two fixed markers for heart disease are being male and having a family history of heart disease.

Describing a risk factor as a "fixed marker" does not mean it is useless or unimportant. Fixed markers can be used to identify those at high risk for an outcome for whom an intervention might be appropriate. For example, low-birth-weight premature children may be targeted for specific interventions to prevent low IQ and poor school performance. Researchers cannot change the fact that these children were born early and small (at least once these children are born), but they can possibly change, by other means, the undesirable outcomes associated with these fixed markers. In addition, identifying fixed markers can often point researchers in the right direction to discover other risk factors that may be implicated in causing and/or preventing the outcome. For example, knowing that gender is a risk factor for a particular disease, researchers might look to hormonal differences or lifestyle differences between men and women to understand why gender is a risk factor and what, other than gender, might be changed to prevent the disease.

What Do We Do with a Risk Factor That Can Change?

We describe risk factors that are not fixed markers—that is, risk factors that can change or be changed—as "variable risk factors."

> *Variable risk factor: A risk factor that can change or be changed.*

Variable risk factors can change spontaneously (such as age or weight) or can be changed by personal choice or medical intervention (such as changing a person's weight with diet or changing a person's blood pressure by administering a drug). Figure 3.1 depicts a flowchart distinguishing fixed markers from variable risk factors.

Consider Example 3.1 describing a variable risk factor.

EXAMPLE 3.1

An article titled "Churchgoers Live Longer, Researchers Find"[2] described how researchers at the University of California at Berkeley found that people who attend church are less likely to die of respiratory or digestive diseases.

The researchers in Example 3.1 demonstrated that whether or not a person attends church is a variable (protective) risk factor for death from respiratory or digestive diseases. Everyone can change whether or not he or she attends church. However, does this result suggest we should encourage people to go to church? If we did, would fewer people die from respiratory or digestive diseases? Simply because a risk factor can change does not mean that changing it will make any difference in preventing (or promoting) the outcome. The result that churchgoers live longer may be an indication of,

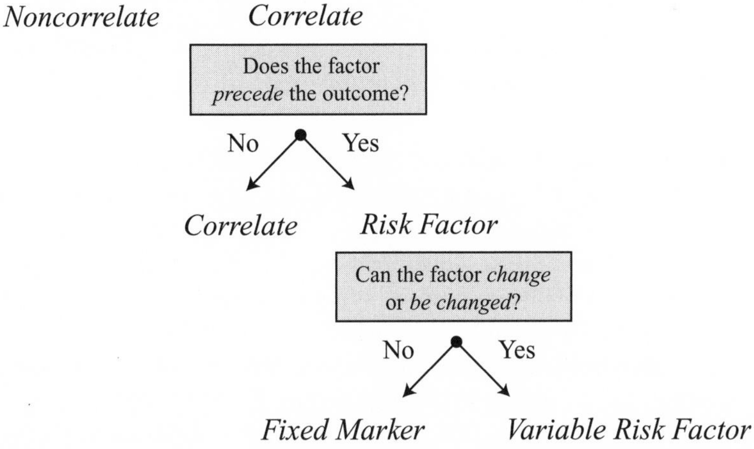

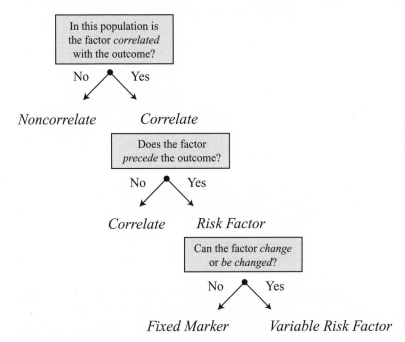

Figure 3.1. A flowchart distinguishing fixed markers from variable risk factors.

for example, the lifestyle, personality, sense of community, or spirituality of people who choose to attend church. More simply, churchgoers may represent a population of people more capable of leaving the house and getting to church. People unable to leave the house because of respiratory or digestive problems are probably also unable to attend church. The description of "variable risk factor" serves as a placeholder until researchers either show that the risk factor is a "variable marker" or a "causal risk factor."

> *Variable marker: A risk factor that can change or be changed, but researchers have not (yet) shown that changing the risk factor alters the risk of the outcome.*
>
> *Causal risk factor: A risk factor that can change and, when changed, has been shown to alter the risk of the outcome.*

The transition between labeling a risk factor a variable marker or a causal risk factor is often a prolonged and rocky one (see Figure 3.2). Labeling a risk factor a causal risk factor requires researchers to show that changing the risk factor changes the risk of the outcome. However, labeling a risk factor a variable marker actually means either researchers are unable to conduct the research to show that changing the risk factor changes the risk of the outcome or they have conducted such research multiple times and so far have been unable to show that changing the risk factor changes the risk of the outcome. Many of the most controversial issues in psychological and medical research and practice are generated at this point. Consider Example 3.2.

EXAMPLE 3.2.

Researchers have shown that couples who live together before they are married are more likely to later get divorced.[3]

Whether or not a couple lives together is a variable risk factor—couples can choose whether or not to live together prior to marriage. However, researchers have not shown that if they persuade a couple who chooses to live together not to (or vice versa, persuade those who choose not to live together to do so), their risk of divorce changes. Whether or not a couple lives together before marriage, for example, may reflect the personalities of people who choose to live together, their religious convictions, or the strength of their relationship, and so forth, and these characteristics, not the act of living together, may lead to divorce. What we don't know is whether the act of living

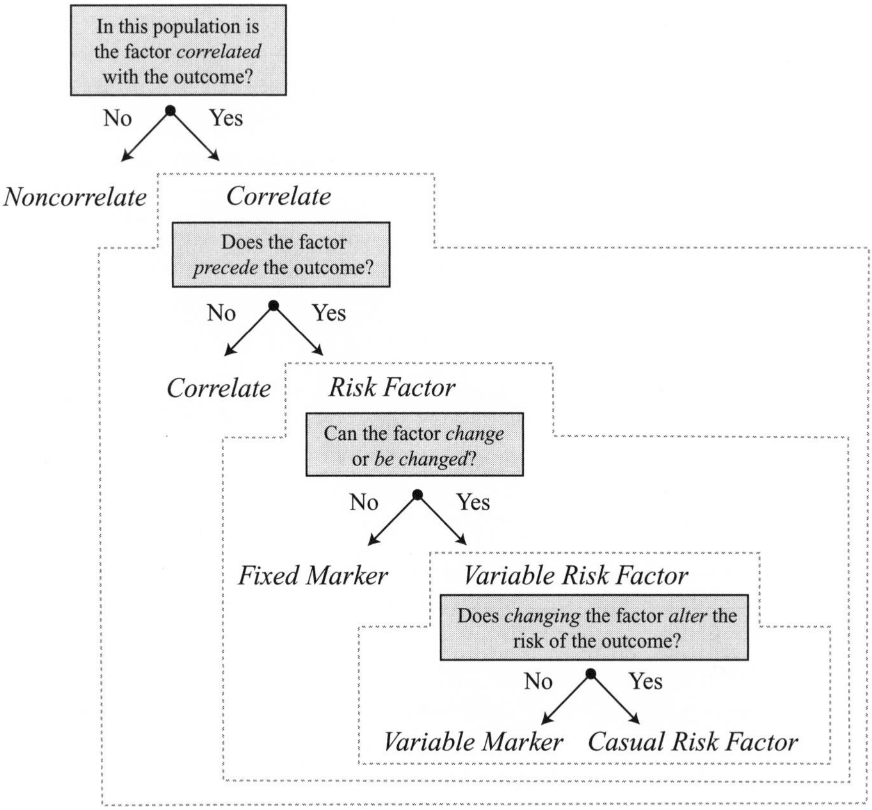

Figure 3.2. A flowchart distinguishing the different types of risk factors.

together prior to marriage in any way directly affects the success of the future marriage.

Consider also Example 3.3, which describes a variable risk factor that the media quickly portrayed as causal.

EXAMPLE 3.3

Researchers at Children's Hospital and Regional Medical Center in Seattle studied whether the number of hours of television young children (ages one and three) watch daily is associated with the risk of attention problems at age seven.[4]

The headlines that followed the report described in Example 3.3 included statements such as "TV May 'Rewire' Children's Brains."[5] Quickly, playground conversations among parents turned to how letting children watch TV *causes* attention problems.

Just as in Example 3.2 about marriage, researchers in Example 3.3 only observed the relationship between TV watching at ages one and three and attention problems at age seven. The authors of the study stated:

> It could be that attentional problems lead to television viewing rather than vice versa. . . . It is also possible that there are characteristics associated with parents who allow their children to watch excessive amounts of television that accounts for the relationship between television viewing and attentional problems. For example, parents who were distracted, neglectful, or otherwise preoccupied might have allowed their children to watch excessive amounts of television in addition to having created a household environment that promoted the development of attentional problems.[4(p712)]

The relationship between TV watching and attention problems described in Example 3.3 has many explanations that don't necessarily indicate causality of TV watching on attention problems. On the other hand, consider another study concerning children watching television that did show that changing the number of hours of television children watched daily changed a different, but also worrisome outcome, obesity, as described in Example 3.4.

EXAMPLE 3.4

Researchers at Stanford University provided an 18-lesson, six-month classroom curriculum devised to reduce television, video, and video game use to volunteer third and fourth graders in a public elementary school in San Jose, California. Researchers then compared the changes in body mass (BMI—a measure of obesity) between students in the school that received the intervention and students from another sociodemographically and scholastically matched public elementary school also in San Jose.[6] While the average BMI increased over the course of the school year for students in both schools, the average increase in BMI among participants at the school where the intervention was provided was smaller than the average increase for participants at the school that had no intervention.

In contrast to the study in Example 3.3, where researchers *observed* that the number of hours of television children watched was associated with the risk of attention problems at age seven, researchers of the study in Example 3.4 demonstrated that *changing* the number of hours of television watched was associated with smaller changes in BMI. One caveat to this result, however, is that the difference in the changes in BMI between the two schools could be due to (unknown) differences in the schools, rather than differences resulting from the change in television viewing habits. Researchers in this study randomly decided which school would receive the intervention, but they did not randomly assign the individual students to whether or not they would receive the intervention. Because the schools were closely matched, most likely the differences were due to television viewing habits, but researchers still cannot completely discount that something about the schools could account for the differences. Thus, this result certainly needs to be corroborated to prove causality, but nevertheless, it does suggest that television watching is a causal risk factor for changes in BMI. In contrast, the result described in Example 3.3 only establishes that television watching at ages one and three is a variable risk factor for attention problems at age seven.

Variable markers and variable risk factors that have not yet been determined to be causal can be used in the same ways as fixed markers: they can identify those at high risk for an outcome and point researchers in the right directions in their quest to find causal risk factors. Risk factors that researchers have demonstrated to be causal can be used just like markers to identify people who are high risk and to identify areas for future research, but they also can be used as a basis of interventions designed to prevent or promote an outcome or can be used by each of us as a reason to make a lifestyle change.

A Causal Risk Factor Is Not Always a Cause

We all want to know exactly what causes particular outcomes. Ideally, we can use this knowledge to prevent or promote those outcomes. Unfortunately, most medical outcomes, such as heart disease and cancer, do not have one single "cause" in the sense that if "the cause" is present, the outcome occurs, and if it is not, the outcome does not occur.

Instead, we focus on causal risk factors—risk factors that can be changed and have been shown to change the risk of the outcomes. Causal risk factors are not necessarily "the cause" of a particular outcome. For example, unprotected sex and sharing of hypodermic needles are causal risk factors for AIDS, but they (alone) do not cause AIDS. The HIV virus *causes* AIDS, but until we can vaccinate against the HIV virus, the only way to prevent AIDS is to change the circumstances and behaviors that lead to the transmission of the HIV virus, that is, changing the causal risk factors. Researchers can show that programs that alter these behaviors reduce the risk of AIDS.

Likewise, because researchers cannot change a genotype, they cannot show that the genotype causes a particular outcome. Few are uncomfortable with labeling gender or race/ethnicity fixed markers, but describing a genotype as a fixed marker rather than a causal risk factor seems more troubling to some. Consider Example 3.5.

EXAMPLE 3.5

Phenylketonuria (PKU) is a genetic metabolic disease in which a single enzyme (phenylalanine hydroxylase) is absent. When this enzyme is absent, the essential amino acid phenylalanine builds up in the blood and can cause mental retardation and other neurological problems. Through adherence to a strict diet, children with PKU can expect normal development and a normal life span.

Children are born with the PKU genotype. The PKU genotype cannot currently be changed and therefore is a fixed marker for PKU retardation. The risk factor for PKU retardation that can change, however, is a person's blood phenylalanine level. When people with PKU avoid phenylalanine in their diet, they can reduce their blood phenylalanine level and sometimes prevent PKU retardation. Thus, the blood phenylalanine level is a causal risk factor for PKU retardation, not the PKU genotype.

In the case of PKU, we understand the temptation to saying PKU retardation is "caused by" an individual's genetic makeup, since evidence indicates that the PKU gene directly encodes an enzyme that leads to abnormal phenylalanine levels that leads to PKU retardation. However, recall that the goal of risk estimation is to discover the causes of diseases and disorders and specifically to develop interventions to prevent them. When a risk factor is unchangeable, such as genotype, race, or ethnicity, researchers can never prove if changing the risk factor changes the risk of the outcome. With respect to PKU, researchers don't know for certain that if they could change the gene, PKU retardation would be prevented. Even though such a conclusion in this case might be true, if they are unable to change the gene, they are no closer to the goal of preventing PKU retardation. In addition, if we are willing to use the word "cause" casually in this case, what prevents us from using "cause" in other cases when the evidence of any causal link is weaker or even nonexistent? By focusing on proven causal risk factors, we are focusing on the risk factors that can potentially prevent or promote an outcome. In other words, we are focusing on things *researchers have shown* we can do something about.

Moreover, another problem with assuming that genetics are causal is that for many diseases such as diabetes, heart disease, and cancer, researchers know that family history is a risk factor but do not yet know which genes are involved or how they operate. In particular, in some cases, the actual direct causal risk factor may be an environmental factor completely unrelated to the genotype. The genotype simply identifies who is susceptible to that environmental factor. We refer to such a gene as a "susceptibility gene," as described in Example 3.6.

EXAMPLE 3.6

An article titled "Study Links Gene to Violence in Boys Who Have Been Abused" describes how researchers followed 442 boys in New Zealand from birth for 26 years. They found that those with a particular genotype who were abused or mistreated were more likely to be aggressive, antisocial, or violent adults than were either those without the genotype (whether or not they were abused) or those with the genotype who were not abused.[7]

The results of the study described in Example 3.6 suggest the genotype determines susceptibility to an environmental risk factor (abuse) but that the genotype itself is not causal. The abuse is the causal risk factor. The genotype only determined for whom that abuse led to aggressive, antisocial, or violent behavior.

How Do Researchers Demonstrate a Risk Factor Is Causal?

Examples 3.2 and 3.3 above, addressing living together before marriage and television watching/attention problems, respectively, illustrate the difficulties researchers face in establishing a risk factor as a causal risk factor. The "gold standard" method to demonstrate a risk factor is causal is a "randomized clinical trial" or RCT, a topic we discuss more thoroughly in Chapter 7. In an RCT, researchers *randomly* assign study participants to either a "treatment" group or a "control" group. Researchers then change a risk factor in the treatment group (by, e.g., administering a drug or placing participants on a particular diet) and leave the risk factor alone in the control group. If the two groups then show different outcomes (assuming the study is well designed and corroborated by other well-designed studies), then researchers have demonstrated that changing the risk factor changes the outcome—that is, that the risk factor is causal.

Part of the controversy in establishing whether or not risk factors are causal has its roots in disagreements about how convincing are "observational" studies, where people are not randomly assigned to treatment or control groups. In observational studies, instead of randomly assigning participants and manipulating risk factors, researchers simply observe behaviors, characteristics, and events and see how they relate to subsequent outcomes of interest. In these studies, the treatment and control groups are usually self-selected—that is, the study participants themselves play some role in determining whether they are in the treatment or control group. For example, in a typical study on the effects of smoking, participants who smoke are compared to participants who do not smoke. The participants themselves, however, made the choice to smoke or not. Other factors that go into determining who will choose to smoke may have just as much to do with any observed differences between a treatment and a control group as does the particular risk factor of interest.

Sometimes researchers will report that they "controlled" for these other factors related to the risk factor of interest (what epidemiologists often refer to as "confounders"). When researchers say they have controlled for other factors, they typically are saying that they used a mathematical model to attempt to estimate and then remove the effects of the other factors (e.g., with respect to living together prior to marriage, researchers looking at divorce might attempt to control for factors such as religion, duration of the relationship, age, etc.) such that the differences between the control and treatment groups can be attributed to the risk factor of interest (e.g., living together prior to marriage). The problem is, researchers have to be aware of all the possible other factors and then they have to correctly model how these other factors influence the outcome. From a statistical point of view, such results can be quite interesting and informative, but they fall far short of proving causality for the risk factor of interest.

Race/ethnicity is a key example of the difficulty in separating a particular risk factor from other related risk factors that may just as well have a greater influence on the outcome as the risk factor of interest. As we pointed out above, race/ethnicity in the United States is a well-established fixed marker for low IQ and other related outcomes of societal concern such as poor school performance and low socioeconomic level. *The Bell Curve* generated great controversy by inappropriately claiming that race "caused" low IQ.[8] *The Bell Curve* was criticized for many reasons, but even at the most trivial level, the authors' conclusions could not be substantiated. Since race is a fixed marker, researchers could not and did not change race to show that it did, indeed, cause low IQ. In Example 3.7, researchers took a different view by recognizing the link between fixed markers such as race and other changeable social disadvantages such as poor health care, poor schooling, poor nutrition, poor child care, and poor parental knowledge and attempted to manipulate these factors to affect IQ.

EXAMPLE 3.7

The Infant Health and Development Program (IHDP), an eight-site study of low-birth-weight premature infants, examined whether intervening to mitigate some social disadvantages resulted in a change in IQ.[9] In an RCT, the parents of children in the treatment group received parental education and support, and the children received high-quality day care. The control group received standard medical care. Children in both groups were closely monitored. At the end of the trial, at three years of age, the treatment group had an average IQ nine points higher than that of the control group. That is, researchers demonstrated that changing some of the *changeable* risk factors associated with low IQ did alter the risk of the outcome of low IQ in this population of low-birth-weight premature infants.

Of course, not every potential causal risk factor can be studied in an RCT. For example, most people accept that smoking is a causal risk factor for lung cancer, but it has never been feasible or ethical to conduct an RCT to "prove" this fact. A researcher cannot randomly assign some people to smoke and others to refrain. However, researchers can randomly assign some smokers to smoking cessation programs and observe whether their risk of lung cancer is different than those smokers not assigned to the smoking cessation program. Researchers can use animal models and show that smoking leads to the same type of lung abnormalities associated with human lung cancer. Researchers can also conduct many different observational studies and control for confounders as best they can. After all these different studies with different flaws with respect to establishing causality, if the evidence from each converges to the same conclusion, at some point we should believe the evidence is convincing enough. The actual point at which such evidence constitutes proof of causality is not a clear one, but it takes much longer and requires more effort than to do a few well-conducted RCTs. In nonrandomized clinical trials, all alternative explanations for the results must be discounted before anyone can conclude causality.

Conclusion and Summary

All risk factors are not equal. Our purpose of classifying the different types of risk factors is to emphasize that although all risk factors can be used to identify those most in need of an intervention and can be used to motivate further research, many, if not most, risk factors cannot be used to prevent or promote an outcome. When we read of an exciting new risk factor, we all need to consider what type that risk factor is before we consider the implications of the finding. Doing otherwise—in particular, assuming a risk factor is necessarily causal—can waste time and money and possibly can harm.

Even when we are convinced that a risk factor is causal, we need to look at other things to decide how much it matters. Often changing a causal risk factor is not a trivial thing. For example, even if we were sure that obesity is a causal risk factor for an untimely death, losing weight is still not an easy thing to do. Or as another example, sometimes taking a drug incurs other undesirable side effects, sometimes even side effects that are worse than the outcome we are trying to prevent. We need to question the value of taking that drug even when it is reasonably effective in preventing or promoting the outcome, and when the effectiveness is low, question even more so. Chapter 4 focuses on how you can tell how much a risk factor matters and ways that researchers can better communicate not only that a new risk factor has been discovered, but also how well that risk factor—and particularly changing that risk factor—predicts the outcome.

- Whether or not a risk factor can change and whether or not changing it changes the likelihood of the outcome are the two criteria distinguishing the different types and uses of risk factors.
- Fixed markers are risk factors that cannot change or be changed. Examples of fixed markers include gender, genotype, location of birth, and race/ethnicity. Because we cannot change fixed markers, they can never be used to alter the risk of the outcome. However, fixed markers can be used to identify those at high risk for an outcome for whom an intervention might be appropriate. Fixed markers can also point researchers in the right direction to discover other risk factors that may be implicated in causing and/or preventing the outcome.
- We describe all risk factors that can change or be changed as "variable risk factors." Examples of variable risk factors include age, weight, level of education, and marital status. Variable risk factors can either be "variable markers" or "causal risk factors."
- A "variable marker" is a risk factor that can change or be changed but researchers have not shown that changing the risk factor alters the risk of the outcome. Variable markers can be used in the same ways as fixed markers.
- A "causal risk factor" is a risk factor that can change and, when changed, has been shown to alter the risk of the outcome. Causal risk factors are the "gold" of risk estimation—they can be used both to

identify those of high risk of the outcome and to provide the bases for interventions to prevent or promote the outcome.

- The most convincing way researchers can demonstrate a risk factor is causal is by a randomized clinical trial (RCT). In an RCT, researchers randomly assign study participants to either a "treatment" group or a "control" group. Researchers manipulate the risk factor in the treatment group (by, e.g., administering a drug or placing participants on a particular diet) and leave the risk factor alone in the control group. If the two groups then show different outcomes (assuming the study is well designed and corroborated by other well-designed studies), then researchers can conclude that changing the risk factor changes the outcome—that is, the risk factor is causal.
- Since not all risk factors and outcomes can be studied in an RCT, researchers can establish causality with "convergence of evidence." Convergence of evidence requires many different studies conducted in many different ways, all converging to the same conclusion. The actual point at which the evidence constitutes proof of causality is not a clear one, but it takes much longer and requires more effort than to do a few well-conducted RCTs.

4

How Do We Know If Something Is an Important Risk Factor?

Statistical and Clinical Significance

If a butterfly flaps its wings in Japan, a hurricane results in Brazil.

This notion, referred to as the "butterfly effect" in chaos theory (and often stated with different locations and different events), is ascribed to MIT mathematician Edward Lorenz. Making fun of his own concept that even tiny relationships among characteristics or events can effect huge changes, Lorenz later joked: "One meteorologist remarked that if the theory were correct, one flap of a seagull's wings would be enough to alter the course of the weather forever."[1]

Joking aside, Lorenz's point is an important one to risk estimation. Some relationship, no matter how small, probably exists between any characteristic and a subsequent event. When a researcher identifies a risk factor—that is, establishes a "statistically significant" relationship between a factor and an outcome and demonstrates the precedence of the factor—the relationship may be so small as to have very little "real-life" significance. Few people would seriously suggest we capture butterflies to prevent unstable weather patterns. Nevertheless, newly discovered risk factors are often taken very seriously, sometimes without much consideration of how well the risk factor actually predicts the outcome.

When pregnant women, for example, hear warnings not to change cats' litter boxes, not to drink alcohol, or not to eat certain fish, unpasteurized cheese, deli meats, or undercooked meats, for example, they rarely also hear how likely it is that failing to heed these warnings will lead to any adverse consequence. Of course, most pregnant women will do anything to protect their unborn child, but what if they make a mistake? Is it possible that the stress from worrying about avoiding all these different activities and foods or worrying about a mistake is more likely to cause adverse consequences than actually doing or eating the wrong thing? Or is it possible that women become immune to so many warnings that they fail to take seriously the ones that really matter?

With these concerns in mind, we hope to attain two related goals in this chapter: to clarify what "statistical significance" means and to clarify how researchers measure and express "clinical significance." We hope to emphasize that even a statistically significant association between a risk factor and an outcome does not necessarily mean that that the relationship is important enough to change personal, medical, or policy decisions.

What Is Statistical Significance?

Two of your coworkers come down with food poisoning. Upon hearing the news, most of us will try to "play detective": What did both eat? And, in particular, did you eat the same thing? Even with less traceable illnesses, from the common cold to cancer, most of us try to find patterns in our knowledge of those afflicted, usually hoping that those same patterns don't hold true for ourselves. Two acquaintances diagnosed with breast cancer, for example, might both be overweight, live near power lines, dye their hair, and have never had children. Both also might drive sport utility vehicles, have brown eyes, enjoy watching football, and vacation in Hawaii. Even if you were to stop dying your hair, move away from power lines, sell your SUV, or skip your Hawaiian vacation, typically little harm would come from such personal "research" based upon what we see around us. However, if you were to publish any such conclusion, particularly if your name, profession, or degree carried some credibility, then your conclusions based on coincidences rather than concrete evidence definitely could harm. For this reason, researchers' first responsibility is to assure that their results are *statistically significant.*

Probably no term has greater importance in research than "statistical significance." If a researcher finds a statistically significant association, then "Eureka!"—a discovery, a publication, possibly more grants! However, a statistically significant result typically means only that the result is unlikely to be due to chance. That is, the researchers collected enough good data to detect a nonrandom association, *no matter how small.*

Statistically significant association: An observed relationship that researchers demonstrate is unlikely to be due to chance.

Recall from Chapter 2 that an association exists between a factor and an outcome when knowing whether or not a person has the outcome (e.g., has had a heart attack) gives you some information about his or her value for the factor (e.g., male or female, cholesterol level) and, alternatively, knowing that person's value of the factor gives you some information about whether or not he or she has the outcome.

In risk estimation, researchers are concerned about the association between certain characteristics or events (potential risk factors) and some subsequent outcome. Demonstrating the existence of such an association is not a simple task. First, researchers must obtain a representative sample from the population, measure both the factor and outcome of interest accurately, select an appropriate test of significance, and correctly apply it. To demonstrate statistical significance, researchers must determine that there is a very small probability that an association as strong as the one observed in the study could have resulted if no relationship in fact existed. By tradition and/or convention, "a very small probability" is usually defined as less than 0.05 (5%) or 0.01 (1%). That is, if there were no relationship and researchers repeated the study 100 times, the result observed in the single study would be expected only five or one of those 100 times. Because five or one out of a hundred is considered "small," researchers conclude that the association is probably nonrandom—that is, some relationship exists between the risk factor and the outcome. The number 0.05 (or 0.01 or whatever significance level is selected before the study is started) is called the "significance level." Often a result is reported as $p < 0.05$ or $p < 0.01$, or $p = 0.049$, or $p = 0.009$. A "p-value" is the estimated probability that a result as strong as that observed in the study would have occurred if there were no relationship between the risk factor and the outcome. Researchers compute the p-value after a study is completed. If the p-value is less than the significance level set before the study began, researchers report the results as "statistically significant."

The Sample Size Influences Whether or Not an Association Is Statistically Significant

To illustrate what goes into determining whether or not a result is statistically significant, consider Example 4.1, a hypothetical example of evaluating whether one drug is better than another.

EXAMPLE 4.1

Suppose researchers randomly assign individuals from a population afflicted with a sometimes fatal disease into two groups. Researchers treat one group (the "old drug" group) with the currently used and approved drug. Researchers give the second group (the "new drug" group) a new experimental drug. Suppose a year later, 50% of the old drug group survived while 100% of the new drug group survived. Is there an association between the choice of drug and the outcome? More specifically, is the new drug better than the old?

Forget statistics for a moment and consider Example 4.1 intuitively. If you were a patient with that disease, would you, on the basis of the data, demand the new drug? Your first question might be: How many people were in each of the two groups?

Suppose there were only two people in each group, and of the four total people, the only one who died was in the old drug group. In this scenario, then, as depicted in Figure 4.1, 50% of the old drug group and 100% of the new drug group survived. Based on this limited sample size, you should be wary of these results. In particular, if researchers added one more person to each group, and of those two new members, the new drug patient died and the old drug patient survived, the survival percentages would now be 67% in each group—a tie between the groups. What a difference one person makes when the sample size is small! If researchers added two more people to each group and both of the new drug patients died but neither of the old drug patients did, then 40% of the new drug group and 80% of the old drug group survives. Now the old drug looks much better. In short, when the sample size is small, adding a few more patients can completely change the results. Consequently, if your own life or well-being were at stake, you should be very skeptical of results based on too small a sample size.

Unfortunately, intuition doesn't usually tell us how many patients are enough. Certainly if the study included 1,000 patients per group with survival rates of 50% in the old drug group and 100% in the new drug group, adding a few more patients to the study, no matter what their outcome, would probably not change the result. If your own life or well-being were at stake, you would probably jump at the chance to use the new drug. But what if instead of 50% versus 100%, the survival rates were 62% in the old drug group and 64% in the new drug group? Even if you could be assured that the new drug had no additional side effects or costs than the old drug, would 1,000 people in each group be large enough to convince you to use the new drug?

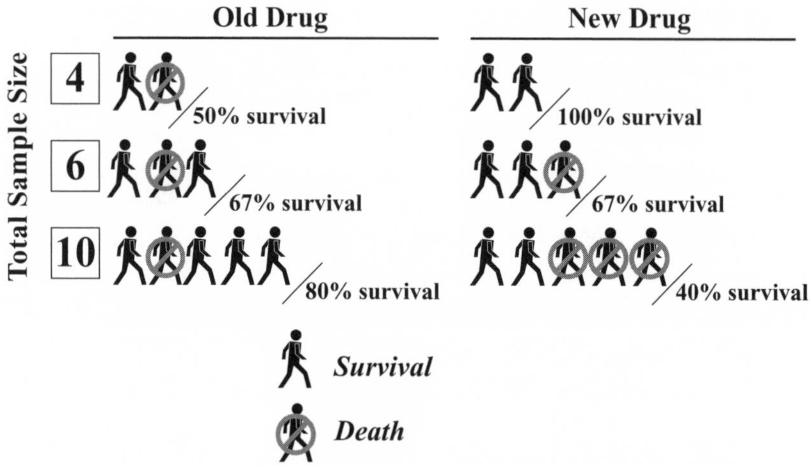

Figure 4.1. How sample size can quickly change whether one drug appears to be better than another. When the sample size is two in each group, and one person dies in the group using the old drug, twice as many people survive using the new drug. Adding just a few people to each group can drastically change which drug "does better."

Intuition plays no role in determining whether something is statistically significant, but some of the same logic principles hold. The sample size (as well as the size of the effect and other indications of the quality of the research) influences both what seems intuitively convincing and what is statistically significant. For a particular association, the greater the sample size, the more likely a result will be "statistically significant." If there is no association, the result will be "statistically significant" 5% or 1% of the time. If there is some association, no matter how small, weak, or trivial it is, researchers will likely achieve a "statistically significant" result when they obtain a large enough sample size.

Consequently, a report of statistical significance should not be taken as a comment on the strength or importance of the association. Instead, a report of statistical significance should be read as a comment on the quality of the evidence and, particularly, as a comment on the sample size. When researchers report a statistically significant result, the very first question they should answer is: How strong is the association? This seems like an obvious first question, but at least in the popular media, the answer is often skipped or obscured. Consider Example 4.2.

EXAMPLE 4.2

In 1984, newspaper headlines reported that a drug, cholestyramine, was found to reduce cardiac events by 19%. These headlines reported the results of a study in which asymptomatic middle-aged men with high cholesterol were randomly assigned to a drug and placebo group and followed for an average of 7.4 years. At the end of that period, researchers reported that 8.6% of the placebo group and 7.0% of the drug group had had a cardiac event. That is, those taking cholestyramine had a 19% lower risk of a cardiac event than those taking a placebo. This was statistically significant at the 5% level (i.e., $p < 0.05$).[2]

Note that this randomized clinical trial (RCT) demonstrated that a high level of cholesterol is a causal risk factor for cardiac events and that use of cholestyramine was a protective factor against cardiac events. That is, as per the definition of a casual risk factor presented in Chapter 3, the study demonstrated that cholesterol level can be changed and, when changed, that the risk of cardiac events was reduced. However, even if cholestyramine is protective, how well does it prevent cardiac events?

This reduction of risk was reported in the newspapers as a 19% decrease in cardiac events. Would you, as a patient, welcome this drug? Would you, as a physician, prescribe this drug? A 19% reduction of risk actually meant that 8.6% of those taking the placebo versus 7.0% of those taking the drug had a cardiac event (the 1.6% difference is 19% of the 8.6% who had cardiac events in the placebo group). The cost of the drug is high, and the seven-year duration of the study is quite a long time. During that time, for an unknown reason, more participants in the drug group died from violent or accidental causes. So this study actually was unable to demonstrate any statistically significant difference in overall death rate. Now, knowing this, would you as a patient welcome this drug? Would you as a physician prescribe this drug? Here, 63 participants would have to take the drug in order to have one less person with a cardiac event than if they had all taken placebo. In other words, doctors treat 62 patients either unnecessarily (they would not have had a cardiac event anyway) or ineffectively (they had a cardiac event anyway) to save one person from having a cardiac event. Considering the costs of the drug and the risk of side effects in the 63 persons, this result may not seem so compelling either to patients or to physicians. The result itself (i.e., how much greater the risk of a cardiac event was in the control group vs. the treatment group) is what matters after statistical significance has been demonstrated, not how statistically significant the result is.

What Does a "Nonstatistically Significant" Result Mean?

"Not statistically significant" means that the evidence collected by the researcher was not sufficient to provide convincing evidence of any association. The sample size may not have been large enough, or something else about the research methods or design might not have been good enough to detect the association that researchers hypothesized existed. A nonstatistically significant result does *not* mean no relationship exists between the potential risk factor and the outcome, only that none was found in this particular study.

For example, returning to the hypothetical Example 4.1, you probably would not conclude that the two drugs were the same if there were only a few study participants in each group and the difference, whether pronounced or not, was not statistically significant. Instead, you should not be convinced one way or the other.

Simply put, nonsignificance is absence of proof, not proof of absence. Unfortunately, interpreting absence of proof as proof of absence is one way people sometimes misconstrue results. Consider Example 4.3.

EXAMPLE 4.3

A *New York Times* headline claims "Study Finds No Link between Breast Cancer and the Pill."[3] Scientists at the Centers for Disease Control and Prevention and the National Institutes of Health surveyed 4,575 women who had breast cancer and 4,682 women who did not. They found that 77% of the cancer patients and 79% of the cancer-free women had taken some type of oral contraceptive.

The study described in Example 4.3 found no statistically significant differences between the cancer patients and the cancer-free women with respect to their use of oral contraceptives. These researchers found no differences, but their result does not mean no differences exist. Many previous studies suggested that use of oral contraceptives is a risk factor for breast cancer, particularly for women with a family history of the disease. When multiple studies find no differences in the risk for breast cancer among women who take and do not take oral contraceptives, then we would be more inclined to believe no real relationship exists between use of oral contraceptives and breast cancer. However, in this case, when results are contradictory, our best strategy is to carefully examine the methods of the different studies to try to understand why the results differ.

When researchers demonstrate a statistically significant relationship between a risk factor and an outcome, they have shown the result is not likely to be a coincidence. To believe a potential risk factor is truly a risk factor, statistical significance is necessary. To believe a potential risk factor is an important risk factor—that is, one we should pay attention to, and if it is causal, we should consider possible actions to change the risk factor—statistical significance is also necessary, but not sufficient. Very small associations between risk factors and outcomes can be statistically significant particularly when researchers collect very large sample sizes. Once researchers demonstrate statistical significance, they need to demonstrate "clinical significance" of the relationship—that is how well does the risk factor predict the outcome?

What Is Clinical Significance?

> *Clinically significant association: An observed relationship that researchers demonstrate matters in some way to medical decision making*

Researchers measure clinical significance typically by indicating the strength of the relationship between the risk factor and the outcome. In general research, the strength of the relationship is called the "effect size," but regarding risk factors, we focus on a particular type of effect size we describe as "potency."

> *Potency: How much better than random—and how much worse than perfect—a risk factor differentiates those who are at high risk for an outcome from those who are at low risk, taking into consideration relevant costs and benefits.*

Potency, as we define it, describes how well the factor predicts the outcome in a very specific way. We focus on potency in terms of how much low- and high-risk groups differ in risk. In Chapter 1 we said that outcomes for risk estimation are always binary. We never said that risk factors have to be binary, such that a risk factor necessarily splits the population into two groups—the high-risk and the low-risk group. However, typically splitting the population into a high-risk and low-risk group is exactly how most people think about and use risk factors. For example, doctors may monitor women with a family history of breast cancer more carefully than they do women without. Doctors may offer blood pressure medication or cholesterol-lowering medication to individuals with cholesterol levels or blood pressure measures exceeding certain thresholds. Medical decision making often necessitates this splitting into two groups—one to treat or intervene with, the other to leave alone. For some risk factors (e.g., cholesterol level or blood pressure), researchers can choose many different ways of defining the high- and low-risk groups.

To illustrate why the potency of a risk factor (causal or not) is so important, consider Example 4.4, an admittedly extreme hypothetical case of how a risk factor might be used to identify who is at highest risk for a disease.

EXAMPLE 4.4

Suppose there is a rapid, deadly disease that, in absence of intervention, afflicts 10% of the population. In addition, suppose an intervention exists that completely prevents the disease but costs $1,000 per person and has fatal side effects for 20% of those treated. Suppose a small city of 10,000 people were to consider four different prevention strategies: no intervention, universal intervention, random intervention, and a "high-risk" intervention strategy. Given what we know about the disease and the intervention, here is what we would expect to happen (also summarized in Table 4.1):

- No intervention: 1,000 people would quickly die of the disease.
- Universal intervention (everyone receives the intervention): No one dies of the disease, but the city spends $10 million and 2,000 people die of the deadly side effects.
- Random intervention (20% of the people are randomly selected for intervention): 800 of the 8,000 untreated people die of the disease, and 400 of the 2,000 treated people die of the fatal side effects. The city spends $2 million, but 1,200 people die.
- "High-risk" intervention (5% of the population have a risk factor; 90% of the people with the risk factor get the disease): The city spends $500,000 to treat 500 high-risk people; 100 of these people die of the deadly side effects, while 6% of the 9,500 untreated people (570 people) die of the disease. [Note: 6% is calculated knowing that the overall risk is 10%.]

Clearly, universal intervention does not make sense in the case described in Example 4.4—the city spends $10 million to increase the number of deaths over what would have happened had they done nothing at all. Even random intervention is worse than no intervention: the city spends $2 million to cause an extra 200 deaths. Only the "high-risk" strategy is

Table 4.1
A Comparison of Four Prevention Strategies for a City of 10,000 People

	No Intervention	Universal Intervention	Random Intervention	"High-Risk" Intervention
Cost ($1,000 per person)	$0	$10 million	$2 million	$500,000
Number of people intervened upon	0	10,000	2,000	500
Number of people for which intervention prevented the disorder	0	1,000	200	450
Number of people intervened upon unnecessarily	0	9,000	1,800	50
Number of deaths from the disorder	1,000	0	800	570
Number of deaths from the intervention	0	2,000	400	100
Total number of deaths	1,000	2,000	1,200	670

better than doing nothing at all—670 people still die, but only 10 of those die because they were treated unnecessarily.

Although this hypothetical example is extreme and used only for illustration, current events have yielded a real example of such a disease and intervention of high concern today: smallpox. Smallpox is a sometimes fatal disease, but a vaccine has been available and had been in use for many years. This vaccine also carries risks, some also fatal. Before the World Health Organization declared smallpox eradicated, children in the United States were routinely vaccinated (universal intervention). As more and more people were vaccinated, the risk that a nonvaccinated person would contract smallpox became smaller and smaller. The reason this routine vaccination ceased in 1972 was essentially because the risk of complications from the vaccine exceeded the perceived risk of contracting the disease.

Today with the threat of bioterrorism, the perceived risk of contracting smallpox has again changed, reigniting the debate about whether the risk of the disease outweighs the risk of serious side effects from the vaccine. Just as in our hypothetical example, if researchers and doctors are going to effectively save lives with respect to small pox or its vaccine, they need to use risk factors to identify who is most likely to contract small pox, as well as use risk factors to identify who is most likely to suffer serious side effects from the vaccine. Health experts have been doing exactly this: persons considered at higher risk of contracting smallpox (e.g., military personnel, health care workers) have been first to be considered for vaccination, while those of higher risk of adverse side effects (e.g., those who are immunocompromised or pregnant or have eczema or heart conditions) have been discouraged from vaccination.

As illustrated both by hypothetical Example 4.4 and the real example of smallpox, the use of risk factors, even just for identification purposes, helps prevent sickness and promote health. These examples also make clear that, typically, randomly selecting who will receive the intervention is a dangerous and expensive strategy. However, when a risk factor fails to do a "good job" at identifying those who would benefit from the intervention, use of the risk factor may not be much better than a random strategy. Hence, we return to why we define potency in terms of how much better than random the risk factor performs. We know that because a risk factor has a statistically significant relationship with the outcome, it will perform better than random. But if it does not perform much better than random, then use of the risk factor to identify who may be at highest risk of the outcome may do more harm and cost more money than doing nothing at all.

How Do Researchers Measure and Communicate Potency?

Unfortunately, researchers measure and communicate potency in many different ways. Researchers from different fields (medicine, epidemiology, psychology, sociology, etc.) contribute to risk estimation, but each of these disciplines uses different standard measures. Few of these measures are mathematically or conceptually simple. Not only do the many different measures make communicating across contributing fields difficult, but also communicating to nonresearchers (policy makers, journalists, anyone who might be interested in the result) is especially difficult since interpreting these measures generally requires experience with the measure as well as some statistical training.

First, consider Example 4.5 illustrating why it is so difficult to convey how much higher the risk is in the high-risk group versus the low-risk group.

EXAMPLE 4.5

Suppose 20% of a particular population will get a disease. Suppose researchers find a risk factor such that 40% of the people in this population who have the risk factor will get the disease. Is this risk factor potent?

At face value, the risk factor described in Example 4.5 appears to be very potent—40% is double the risk of 20%. However, there are other considerations that might call into question the usefulness of this risk factor. First, what percentage of the population has the risk factor? If 50% of the population has the risk factor, then the other 50% of the population has 0% risk of the outcome. A risk factor that can eliminate half the population from consideration is probably a very potent risk factor, but what if the intervention proposed for the 50% with the risk factor has dangerous side effects? Then half the population will be exposed to a dangerous intervention when only 40% will get the disease the intervention is attempting to prevent.

On the other hand, suppose only 10% of the population has the risk factor. Then a dangerous intervention would at least not affect as many people, but the 90% of the population without the risk factor still has an 18% risk of the disease. The risk factor did not do much to help lower the risk in the general population.

Ultimately, determining whether a risk factor is potent comes down to the basic issue of how should researchers trade off *false positives*—saying someone is high risk of the outcome when they will *not* have the outcome—and *false negatives*—saying someone is low risk for the outcome when they *will* have the outcome? In the case of disease prevention, a false positive may result in providing an intervention to someone who would not have otherwise contracted the disease, while a false negative will result in failing to provide the intervention to someone who will contract the disease. When the outcome is, for example, contracting a cold, either type of mistake in prediction is not too worrisome. On the other hand, when the outcome is cardiac death, being identified as "high risk" allows an individual to make lifestyle changes to prevent the outcome. However, being misidentified as "high risk" may create problems, particularly if those lifestyle changes include, for example, a drug intervention that may have side effects. With respect to the prostate-specific antigen (PSA) test to prevent morbidity and mortality from prostate cancer, being misidentified as low risk might mean a potentially deadly cancer goes undetected (one study estimated that among men over the age of 62, 15% of men with a PSA level less than 4.0 ng/ml may still have prostate cancer[4]). On the other hand, being misidentified as high risk might lead to a biopsy and the detection of a potentially harmless prostate cancer. The treatment for that harmless prostate cancer might include surgeries that could leave the man impotent and incontinent.

The many different measures of potency exist because each represents a different way to measure how much better than random and/or how much worse than perfect a risk factor performs, and specifically, each measure trades off the problems of false positives versus false negatives in a different way. Unfortunately, typically the same potency measure is used within a particular discipline (e.g., the "odds ratio" in epidemiology, "gamma" in sociology, "phi coefficient" and "kappa coefficient" in psychology), even though the problems of false positives versus false negatives are different for different risk factors, different outcomes, and different populations.

We mention the names of some of the different measures here only to emphasize the difficulty in communicating and understanding results when so many different measures are used by different researchers. In some cases, some of these measures can indicate the risk factor is potent, while another measure calculated for the same risk factor, same population, and same outcome might indicate the risk factor is not potent at all.

If communicating potency is a challenge among researchers, with what measure should the nonresearcher (policy makers, journalists, anyone trying to get information from a research result) become familiar to understand the research results? Chapter 9 includes a comprehensive discussion of many different measures of potency, as well as our recommendation for the best measure of potency for scientific applications (the weighted kappa coefficient). For this discussion, however, it is not necessary to be familiar with these different measures, but rather to recognize the difficulty in measuring potency and the greater difficulty in communicating and understanding it, particularly when even the researchers do not agree. When using the weighted kappa coefficient, researchers select a weight to reflect how important it is to avoid false positives versus avoiding false negatives. Then a kappa of 0 indicates random association, a kappa of 1 indicates perfect association, and a kappa somewhere in between indicates how far between random and perfect the association is, given the stated relative importance of false positives versus false negatives. However, for communication to the general public, we suggest, instead, another potency measure related to the weighted kappa that is easier to understand and facilitates taking personal views of the relative importance of false positives and false negatives into account.

How Could Researchers Communicate Clinical Significance in a Way Easier for Everyone to Comprehend?

For widespread communication with everyone, we recommend a potency measure we call "number needed to treat/take," or NNT.

> *Number needed to treat/take (NNT): The number of people that must be selected from each of the "high-risk" and the "low-risk" groups such that we can expect the high-risk group to have one more occurrence of the outcome than the low-risk group. Mathematically, NNT = 1/[risk(high risk) – risk(low risk)]. By "risk(high risk)" or "risk(low risk)," we mean the probability that someone in the high- or low-risk groups will have the outcome.*

We actually used NNT in discussing Example 4.2 when we said that doctors would have to treat 63 patients with cholestyramine to prevent one person from having a cardiac event. That is, if researchers selected 63 participants from the control group and 63 patients from the treatment group (i.e., those who took cholestyramine), researchers would expect 4.4 people to have cardiac events in the control group and 5.4 people to have cardiac events in the treatment group—a difference of one person [8.6% of the control group and 7.0% of the treatment group had a cardiac event; the risk in the treatment group is 8.6%, and the risk in the control group is 7%; NNT is then 1/(0.086 – 0.07) = 63].

NNT originally comes from the RCT arena and is typically referred to as "number needed to treat" (with, e.g., cholestyramine). So that NNT applies to all risk factors—even those that are not treatments—we will also refer to NNT as "number needed to take," preserving the abbreviation NNT. NNT could apply to, for example, how many women and how many men that researchers would have to select to expect one more of the women than of the men to be diagnosed with depression within the next year.

A small NNT indicates that the risk factor is very potent—that is, researchers do not need to look at too many people from each of the high- and low-risk groups to see a difference in the number of people who will have the outcome. In fact, when the NNT is 1, the risk factor perfectly predicts who will have the outcome and who will not because if researchers select one person from the high-risk group and one person from the low-risk group, they will always have one more occurrence of the outcome in the high-risk group—that is, the one person from the high-risk group will have the outcome, and the one from the low-risk group will not.

Another way of looking at NNT when doctors intend to treat the high-risk people is to consider what happens if they treat NNT people. Then, NNT – 1 people will be treated unnecessarily and possibly harmed, depending on the treatment. When the NNT is 1, no one will be treated unnecessarily. When the NNT is large, many people will be treated unnecessarily.

To see how we might think about NNT, consider Example 4.6.

EXAMPLE 4.6

The collaborative group on Hormone Factors in Breast Cancer reanalyzed 47 epidemiological studies and reported finding that breast-feeding is a protective factor against breast cancer. The *San Jose Mercury News* article describing these results, titled "Study: Breast-feeding Reduces Cancer,"[5] indicated that in the United States, a woman's average current lifetime risk of developing breast cancer is about 12.5%. An additional year of breast-feeding they estimate would lower the lifetime risk to about 12%.

If we look at the numbers in Example 4.6 from an NNT standpoint, the risk in the high-risk group (i.e., those who do not breast-feed an additional year) is 12.5%, and the risk in the low-risk group (i.e., those who breast-feed an additional year) is 12%. Then, NNT = 1/(0.125 – 0.120) = 200. Two hundred women would have to breast-feed an additional year to have one less case of breast cancer than if those 200 women had not breast-fed that additional year. That means that, at the very least, 199 women would have to breast-feed an additional year unnecessarily or ineffectively (with respect to breast cancer) for one woman to avoid breast cancer. If we were considering urging women to breast-feed an additional year to reduce the incidence of breast cancer, we would have to consider the effect on the 199 women relative to the benefit to the one.

For a "treatment" that is expensive and/or dangerous, NNT should be quite small. For example, in Example 4.6, the "treatment" is breast-feeding—not usually an expensive or dangerous treatment. In fact, there are many other documented benefits of breast-feeding for both the mother and child other than cancer prevention. Thus, NNT = 200 in this case might be quite acceptable. On the other hand, suppose 200 women needed to have a new type of surgery to prevent one case of breast cancer? What if that surgery were a radical mastectomy? What if we are talking about similar numbers for prostate surgeries for men?

Because we are all medical decision makers in terms of our own and our family's health, interpreting NNTs is somewhat of a subjective and individual endeavor. Above we said that an NNT of 200 for breast-feeding to prevent breast cancer "might be" quite acceptable while asking whether it would be acceptable for surgery, or even radical mastectomies. In reality, whether or not 200 is large or small depends on who is considering breast-feeding or having surgery or whatever the treatment and outcome under consideration is. Breast-feeding is easy for some, difficult for others, and downright dangerous for yet others (e.g., HIV-positive mothers). The individual or at least the physician needs to consider the particular situation. Nevertheless, NNT provides a way for everyone, even without a statistical background, to evaluate, at least subjectively, how much a risk factor matters to them.

Recently, more and more studies are beginning to provide potency measures similar to NNT. For example, the principal results from the Women's Health Initiative's RCT that tested whether hormone replacement therapy (HRT) was associated with higher or lower risks of various cancers, coronary heart disease (CHD), and other diseases included the following summary: "Over 1 year, 10,000 women taking estrogen plus progestin compared with placebo might experience 7 more CHD events, 8 more strokes, 8 more PEs [pulmonary embolisms], 8 more invasive breast cancers, 6 fewer colorectal cancers, and 5 fewer hip fractures. Combining all the monitored outcomes, women taking estrogen plus progestin might expect 19 more events per year per 10,000 women than women taking placebo."[6(p331)]

Although these measures presented by the Women's Health Initiative are not exactly NNT, they do provide an indication comprehensible to most nonresearchers of how much taking this particular form of HRT changes the risks of the outcomes such as breast cancer and heart attacks. Perhaps women who were taking HRT only because they believed HRT was *protective* against heart disease would be motivated by such potency measures to stop taking

HRT. On the other hand, women whose lives have been impaired because of their extreme symptoms of menopause might be encouraged by these potency measures because the number of adverse events per 10,000 women is not extremely high.

Conclusion and Summary

NNT, as is any other measure of potency, is one way to move past statistical significance toward clinical significance. We think it is an excellent measure to report, particularly in the popular media, because it is one measure of potency easy for the nonresearcher to comprehend, and it fosters the necessary contemplation about the relative importance of false positives and false negatives. Nevertheless, the message this chapter hopes to convey is that researchers must always take some step beyond statistical significance to communicate why the finding matters. In Chapter 9, we discuss at greater length the different "steps" researchers can take to communicate the importance, or lack thereof, of statistically significant results. To conclude this chapter, however, we return to our theme of urging the necessity of clear and correct communication to risk research. Communicating clinical significance in a way that is more understandable to everyone is simply another vital step to changing the face of risk research.

Still, often individual risk factors—even very important ones to medical decision making—do not alone have high potency. However, when considered in conjunction with other risk factors, the combination of risk factors does a much better job in predicting whether or not someone will have the outcome. Often the consideration of multiple risk factors can be a very confusing undertaking. How do we respond when we have some, but not all, risk factors for a particular outcome? In Chapter 5 we hope to reduce some of that confusion by discussing ways in which risk factors work together to produce an outcome.

- Researchers' first responsibility is to ensure that their results are statistically significant.
- A statistically significant association is an observed relationship that researchers demonstrate is unlikely to be due to chance.
- To demonstrate statistical significance, the researcher must show that there is a very small probability that an association as strong as the one observed in the study could have resulted if no relationship, in fact, existed.
- The number of people included in a study (the "sample size") has a great influence on whether or not an association is statistically

significant. If a study does not include enough people, a relationship that looks strong and real may not be statistically significant. On the other hand, if a study includes very many people, even a very small relationship may be statistically significant.

- A nonstatistically significant result does not prove there is no association. It only means the data collected do not provide convincing evidence that an association exists.
- Even results that are statistically significant may not be significant at all from a practical point of view. Once researchers have demonstrated that the result is statistically significant, they need to demonstrate how clinically significant it is.
- A "clinically significant association" is an observed relationship that researchers demonstrate is relevant in some way to medical decision making. Researchers measure clinical significance typically by indicating the strength of the relationship between the risk factor and the outcome. In general research, the strength of the relationship is called the "effect size," but with respect to risk factors, we focus on a particular type of effect size we describe as "potency."
- Potency describes how much better than random—and how much worse than perfect—a risk factor differentiates those who are high risk for an outcome versus those who are low risk, taking into consideration relevant costs and benefits.
- Currently, there are many different available and used measures of potency. Selecting the most appropriate measure of potency for a particular risk factor and outcome depends on considering the relative importance of correctly identifying those who will have the outcome and correctly identifying those who will not have the outcome.
- For clinical or policy communication, we recommend reporting the "number needed to treat/take" (NNT). For the purposes of risk estimation, NNT is the number of people that must be selected from each of the "high-risk" and the "low-risk" groups such that we can expect the high-risk group to have one more occurrence of the outcome than the low-risk group. The smaller the NNT, the more potent the risk factor. The larger the NNT, the weaker the risk factor. If an intervention or treatment were to be administered to NNT people, NNT – 1 people would be treated unnecessarily. An NNT of 1 means no one would be treated unnecessarily, while a large NNT indicates many people would be treated unnecessarily. Thus, evaluating an NNT requires trading off the possible harm to NNT – 1 people against the benefit to the one person.

5

How Do Risk Factors Work Together? Moderators, Mediators, and Other "Inter-actions"

> "I don't know anybody who doesn't think the government might not have done it," Cleve confided.
>
> By now, there were lots of theories and Cleve had heard them all. In New York, the epidemic seemed to snipe vengefully at the top of Manhattan's ziggurat of beauty. People called it the "Saint's disease" because everybody who got it seemed to be among the guys who danced all night at that popular disco. Maybe they put something in the drinks, the water, the air. In San Francisco, the epidemic spread first through the leather scene. Gay men began suspiciously eyeing barroom ionizers that helped eliminate cigarette smoke. Maybe those gadgets were emitting something else, something deadly.
>
> —From *And the Band Played On,* Randy Shilts's powerful description of the early days of the AIDS epidemic

When the only known risk factor for AIDS was homosexuality, the theory that the government was responsible was probably as plausible as any other explanation. The mysterious way in which AIDS suddenly began killing gay men understandably could have led to such suspicions. Now that researchers have identified the HIV virus and its modes of transmission, we have moved beyond suspicions and know how to prevent and delay the course of the disease. Ideally at some point in our lifetimes, we will witness the discovery of a vaccination or a cure.

Even though the process of identifying HIV that Randy Shilts describes[1(p149)] was chaotic, how researchers identify the paths leading to a disorder caused by an organism is relatively straightforward. Identifying such paths for complex disorders, such as cancer, heart disease, diabetes, Alzheimer's disease, depression, or schizophrenia, is much more difficult since these disorders probably have many different causes, some working together and acting in different ways for different people. For such disorders, researchers can easily identify multiple risk factors. But how should we think about and respond to a long list of risk factors? Specifically, does having multiple risk factors put us at greater risk than having only one or two? Can risk factors cancel each other out? If, for example, we have light-colored eyes and had a lot of past sun exposure, but we also have dark skin and dark hair, are we less or more at risk for skin cancer than others with little previous sun exposure or someone whose skin, hair, and eye color are different? How can we "put together" our knowledge of multiple risk factors?

The answers to such questions are difficult to find because such questions are, to date, not well addressed in risk research. Typically, the more research conducted on a particular disease or disorder, the longer the list of risk factors identified. These risk factors are piled up or researchers count or average them, but such strategies seldom help increase our understanding of the chain of events that might lead to an outcome or how different combinations of risk factors might affect how likely someone is to eventually have the outcome. Often, each of these individual risk factors, taken alone, has little clinical significance—that is, has low potency. Considered together, they may do a much better job at describing who is at high risk and who is at low risk. However, how should they be considered together?

In this chapter, we introduce the ways in which two risk factors work together to predict an outcome. We will call these "inter-actions" because they describe the actions between or among risk factors for the same outcome. The word "interaction" typically has a statistical connotation that is more limited than what we mean here. Thus, we include a hyphen to differentiate "inter-action" from the statistical term "interaction."

Why Should We Care about Inter-actions?

In this chapter, we describe inter-actions such as moderators and mediators—two terms originally defined by Baron and Kenney[2] and in frequent use by researchers. We also describe and define three other inter-actions that complete the possible ways that two risk factors might work together: proxy, overlapping, and independent.[3]

These descriptors of risk factors are different from the ones we defined in preceding chapters, such as fixed marker, variable risk factor, and causal risk factor—those terms apply to a *single* risk factor with reference to an outcome in a population. Inter-actions, on the other hand, apply to a *pair* of risk factors with reference to an outcome in a population and can be extended to connect more than two risk factors to the outcome. By linking risk factors together in this way, researchers can sort out important from unnecessary or redundant risk factors and move closer to understanding the crucial core set of risk factors and how they work together.

For the nonresearcher, a basic understanding of these relationships provides a framework for considering and processing those long laundry lists of risk factors we often come across for most diseases or disorders. For example, the American Academy of Family Physicians published the following list of 16 risk factors for osteoporosis: female gender, petite body frame, white ancestry, Asian ancestry, sedentary lifestyle/immobilization, nulliparity (no pregnancies), increasing age, high caffeine intake, renal disease, lifelong low calcium intake, smoking, excessive alcohol use, long-term use of certain drugs, postmenopausal status, low body weight, and impaired calcium absorption.[4] Just by inspection, we may suspect that many of these risk factors are redundant in some way (e.g., postmenopausal status, female gender, and increasing age), and perhaps some lead to others (e.g., maybe long-term use of certain drugs, smoking, or excessive alcohol use leads to impaired calcium absorption). Since some of these risk factors apply only to women (e.g., nulliparity and postmenopausal status), if we are male do we just ignore these and assume the rest still apply? If researchers could sort out these risk factors for us, we would have a start in understanding our risk for a particular disease or disorder. But even in absence of that, understanding how different risk factors may work together is a useful tool for looking critically at such long lists of risk factors.

As we present the five inter-actions in this chapter, we include two coordinated sets of definitions for each term: a conceptual definition and an operational definition. The conceptual definitions explain how risk factors work together—the most important aspect for the nonresearcher to be aware of in order to understand how multiple risk factors might interrelate. However, from the researcher's point of view, such a definition is too imprecise. Hence, the operational definition clearly differentiates the inter-actions by providing the exact "rules" for researchers to demonstrate such an inter-action exists.

What Is a Proxy Risk Factor?

We begin with a proxy risk factor, in part because it is the easiest inter-action to explain and comprehend. Moreover, proxy risk factors also are the root of many misleading and confusing statements about risk.

Proxy risk factor: A risk factor that is a risk factor for an outcome only because it is strongly associated with another, more relevant, risk factor.

Consider Example 5.1.

EXAMPLE 5.1

Suppose researchers identified two risk factors for teen-onset depression: gender (girls are *more likely* to have teen-onset depression) and ball-throwing ability at age 10 (kids who throw farther are *less likely* to have teen-onset depression). Should an intervention be designed to see if improving ball-throwing ability reduces the likelihood of teen-onset depression?

After reading Chapter 3 on causality, to the question in Example 5.1 we should answer, "No, researchers did not demonstrate that ball-throwing ability is a causal risk factor." Nevertheless, since ball-throwing ability is changeable, researchers could conceivably take the time and money to attempt to demonstrate its causality. However, before taking such a step, researchers would probably recognize the relationship between gender and ball-throwing ability. At age 10, boys are probably more likely to throw a ball farther than are girls. Boys are also less likely to have teen-onset depression. Ball-throwing ability probably appears to be protective against teen-onset depression only because being male is protective against teen-onset depression. Girls who throw a ball farther are probably not less likely to become depressed than are girls who do not, and the same is probably true of boys. In this case, we would describe ball-throwing ability as a proxy to gender. That is, ball-throwing ability is a risk factor for teen-onset depression only because of its relationship to gender, a true risk factor for teenage depression.

Operationally, researchers can identify that a risk factor, such as ball-throwing ability, is acting as a proxy to more relevant risk factor, such as gender, if (1) the two risk factors are correlated, (2) neither risk factor precedes the other *or* the more relevant risk factor precedes the proxy, and (3) when researchers attempt to use both risk factors to predict the outcome, only the more relevant risk factor matters.[3] We discuss this last requirement in more depth in Chapter 10, where we return to exactly how researchers identify the five inter-actions. However, what is important here is that a proxy risk factor does not improve our ability to predict the outcome when we already know about the other risk factor—just as knowing how far a child can throw a ball does not help us better predict whether he or she will have teen-onset depression when we already know that child's gender. If we do not know the child's gender, then ball-throwing ability might help, but if we do, ball-throwing ability is simply a superfluous piece of information. Thus, ball-throwing ability is a risk factor for teen-onset depression only because of the information it conveys about gender.

Another way to think about and remember the definition of a proxy risk factor is to consider a path analogy—an analogy that coincides well with researchers' goal of identifying causal pathways to an outcome. A proxy risk factor is like a side road of a direct route to a destination. The more relevant risk factor is the direct route. As Figure 5.1 illustrates, you may find yourself on the side road because you are lost, you need to run an errand or to rest, or even just for scenic interest, but the only way to your destination (i.e., the outcome) is to return to the direct route.

When researchers find that a risk factor is proxy to another risk factor, they should set it aside in order to focus on the other risk factor. This isn't to say that proxies are not risk factors, and sometimes even important risk factors. In fact, in cases when a risk factor cannot be measured, the proxies of that risk factor may be the only risk factors researchers can study. But when the risk factor is available, considering its proxies simultaneously detracts from the really important risk factors. Imagine the confusion if the directions from starting point to destination included all side roads, giving them equal

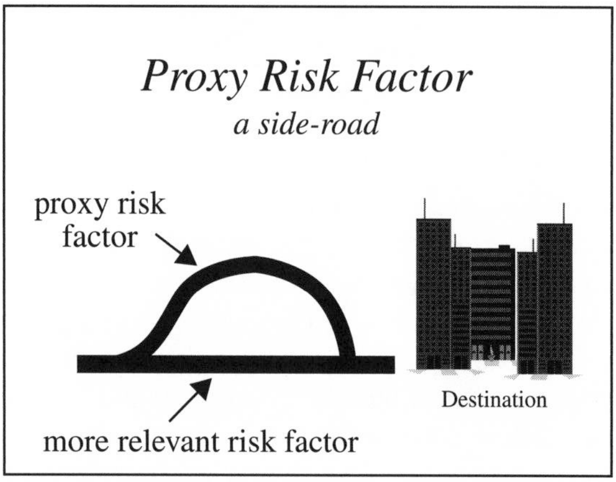

Figure 5.1. An illustrated analogy between a proxy risk factor and a side road.

importance to the direct highway leading from the starting point to the destination.

Some of the risk factors we have already discussed may actually be proxy risk factors to other risk factors. For example, in that long list of 16 risk factors for osteoporosis, perhaps petite body frame is proxy to low body weight, or low body weight is proxy to petite body frame. Or consider Example 5.2, which we presented before concerning church attendance.

EXAMPLE 5.2

An article titled "Churchgoers Live Longer, Researchers Find"[5] describes how researchers at the University of California at Berkeley found that people who attend church are less likely to die of respiratory or digestive diseases.

We have already discussed alternative explanations for this result, other than the explanation that attending church prevents people from dying of respiratory or digestive diseases. Many of these explanations suggest that church attendance might be proxy to another risk factor. For example, attending church could be a proxy to spirituality. Or perhaps attending church is proxy for having a social support network. Or even more simply, attending church could be an indication of being physically able to leave the house and go to church. Perhaps the same individuals who are ailing and unable to attend church are also more likely to develop respiratory and digestive diseases.

We are only speculating about the possible reasons for the result. In fact, we could be wrong. Church attendance could be the protective factor, and when considered simultaneously with spirituality, social support, and physical ability, only church attendance matters. A researcher can discern which is the case by applying the operational definition of a proxy risk factor to a data set containing all four potential risk factors.

Researchers cannot easily prove that a particular risk factor is *not* a proxy to another unknown and unidentified risk factor. Thus, any risk factor needs to be considered from many different angles before it can be taken too seriously. More important, when researchers simultaneously consider many risk factors for the same outcome, they must try to weed out the proxy risk factors and focus on the ones that matter most. Moreover, when nonresearchers examine a laundry list of risk factors for an outcome, they should consider whether some of these might be proxies and demand more information from the researchers before becoming inundated with superfluous information.

What Is an Overlapping Risk Factor?

An overlapping risk factor is similar to a proxy risk factor in that it is closely related to another risk factor. However, whereas researchers should identify and set aside proxy risk factors, they should combine overlapping risk factors to create a single risk factor.

> *Overlapping risk factors: Risk factors for the same outcome that are partially or wholly redundant to each other—they either measure the same "thing" in different ways or they are simply two different names for the same "thing."*

For example, in that list of 16 risk factors for osteoporosis, several of the risk factors could be overlapping. Five of the risk factors (sedentary lifestyle/immobilization, high caffeine intake, smoking, excessive alcohol use, and long-term use of certain drugs) might all reflect poor health habits. Perhaps some or all of them are overlapping in some way? Or perhaps some are proxy to others? Researchers can identify whether each pair of these risk factors has a proxy or an overlapping relationship by applying the operational definitions. Risk factors are overlapping if (1) they are correlated, (2) neither risk factor precedes the other, and (3) when researchers attempt to use both risk factors to predict the outcome, both risk factors matter.[3]

For example, smoking and alcohol use are generally correlated. There is no clear time precedence between the two. If researchers found that smoking and alcohol use together predicted osteoporosis better than either alone, then they are overlapping risk factors for osteoporosis. In this case, researchers might consider defining a factor that would include smoking, alcohol use, and perhaps other associated poor health habits.

As another example, in 1989 right after the Loma Prieta earthquake in the San Francisco Bay Area, newscasters reported that overpasses on Highway 17, Highway 880, and the Nimitz Freeway had collapsed. Those not familiar with the Bay Area probably counted that as three collapses; those familiar with the Bay Area were more likely to correctly count one, because Highway 17, Highway 880, and the Nimitz Freeway were three names often used to refer to the same highway.

Although this Loma Prieta example does not describe risk factors, it does describe how double and triple counting can occur and cause confusion when the same thing has different names. In the path analogy, overlapping risk factors are the same road with multiple names or different lanes of the same road. When two risk factors are perfectly overlapping (e.g., weight in pounds and weight in kilograms), which risk factor we pay attention to doesn't matter: we're still traveling on the same road. We would be less likely to be confused, however, if we know the roads are one and the same. Two risk factors that are not perfectly overlapping (such as weight in pounds and waist circumference) are like two different lanes of the same road (see Figure 5.2). You will typically use more than one lane of the same road to get to your destination most efficiently, but if you were to give directions to the destination, you will only describe the one road. Similarly, combining overlapping risk factors creates a more potent risk factor than either risk factor alone. For example, researchers can consider the information given by weight in pounds and waist circumference jointly by using some general indication of adiposity ("fatness") such as body mass index (BMI) or percent body fat. The dangers of considering two overlapping risk factors simultaneously without combining them is similar to driving in both lanes at the same time or the increased fear of hearing three highway overpasses collapsed in the Bay Area rather than one. It is simply confusing and misleading and maybe even dangerous.

Consider Example 5.3, which describes overlapping risk factors.

EXAMPLE 5.3

When people are depressed, they are often anxious. Conversely, when they are anxious, they are often depressed. Consequently, a measure of depression and a measure of anxiety may be overlapping risk factors for an outcome, such as a subsequent suicide attempt.

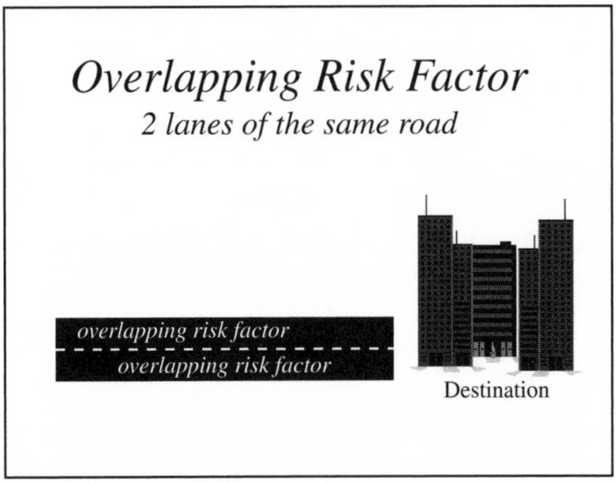

Figure 5.2. An illustrated analogy between an overlapping risk factor and a road with two lanes or two names.

In Example 5.3, if depression and anxiety were overlapping risk factors for a subsequent suicide attempt, then measures of depression and anxiety taken at the same time would be correlated with one another and, together, would better predict whether or not a person attempts suicide than would either measure alone. One interpretation for such a result would be that measures of depression and anxiety actually represent the same underlying "negative affect" that may lead to a suicide attempt, and combining them may represent a better measure of that negative affect than using either one alone.

What Is a Moderator?

In everyday language, the word "moderator" means a person who presides over a meeting or a debate and perhaps monitors and directs its progress. For risk estimation, we use the term moderator to describe a risk factor that "presides" over another risk factor by specifying in whom or under what conditions that other risk factor will affect the outcome. Specifically, depending on the value of the moderator—for example, depending upon whether the individual is male or female—the relationship of another risk factor and the outcome is different.

> *Moderator: A risk factor that can be used to divide the population into groups such that within those groups, another risk factor for the same outcome operates differently.*

We have already alluded to several moderator relationships, particularly in Chapter 2, where we discussed how risk factors often are different within different populations—for example, among men and women, among children and adults, or among different racial groups. Moderators are very likely common but unrecognized, because the unfortunate tendency of research of the past was to assume that research done on one population (e.g., men) was applicable to others (e.g., women or children).

Consider Example 5.4 about genes, child abuse, and subsequent adult violence, which we discussed in Chapter 3:

EXAMPLE 5.4

An article titled "Study Links Gene to Violence in Boys Who Have Been Abused" describes how researchers followed 442 boys in New Zealand from birth for 26 years. They found that those with a particular genotype who were abused or mistreated were more likely to be aggressive, antisocial, or violent adults than either those without the genotype (whether or not they were abused) or those with the genotype who were not abused.[6]

When we introduced this example in Chapter 3 (Example 3.6), we described the genotype as a "susceptibility" gene: those with the gene were more susceptible to become violent as adults if they were abused as children. In this case, the genotype moderates the effect of abuse on subsequent adult violence. That is, if we split the population into two groups, those with the genotype and those without, we see that the role abuse plays relative to the outcome is different in the two groups.

Operationally, researchers can identify a moderator if (1) the two risk factors are uncorrelated, (2) the moderator precedes the other risk factor, and (3) within the subgroups defined by the moderator, the potency of the other risk factor is different.

In our path analogy, a moderator is a "fork in the road" that dictates who goes right and who goes left (see Figure 5.3). The "right" and "left" routes are different. A common "fork" is gender: often the risk factors for a disease influence the outcome differently among men and women. Similarly, race and/or ethnicity also is a common "fork," for example, the different rates and progression of cancer, heart disease, and diabetes among Asians compared with the general U.S. population.[7] Gender and race both appear in the list of 16 risk factors for osteoporosis, and particularly since some of the risk factors listed only apply to women, one or both of these risk factors might moderate the effects of others with respect to osteoporosis.

Consider Example 5.5, which describes a classic case of a moderator relationship and of primary importance in medical research.

EXAMPLE 5.5

An article titled "Breast-Cancer Study Finds Chemotherapy Not for All"[8] describes how a team of researchers from nine countries reported that postmenopausal women with hormone-sensitive breast cancer that had not spread to the lymph nodes received no benefit from chemotherapy. Instead, after surgery, the estrogen-blocking drug tamoxifen was protective against continued growth of the cancer. In addition, they found that for postmenopausal women whose breast cancer was not hormone sensitive, chemotherapy followed by tamoxifen offered the most benefit.

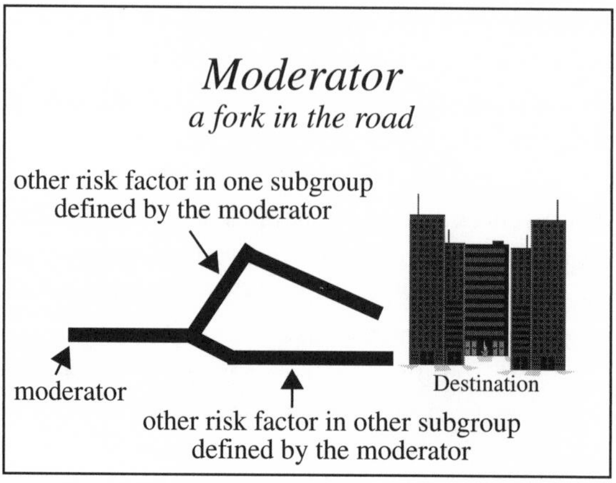

Figure 5.3. An illustrated analogy between a moderator and a fork in the road. Along the different paths defined by the moderator, the other moderated risk factor operates differently.

What researchers probably saw in the study described in Example 5.5 is that both the treatment choice and whether or not the woman had hormone-sensitive breast cancer that had not spread to the lymph nodes were risk factors for whether or not the cancer went into remission. The key finding, however, was the relationship between the two risk factors—specifically, that whether or not the cancer was hormone sensitive and had spread to the lymph nodes moderated the effect of the treatment. Among those whose breast cancer was *not* hormone sensitive and had *not* spread to the lymph nodes, chemotherapy increased the likelihood that the cancer went into remission, while among those whose breast cancer was hormone sensitive, chemotherapy did not change that likelihood.

Identifying the moderator allows researchers to explore different treatment options for different subpopulations defined by the moderator and to optimize the treatment for each subpopulation. This particular result suggests that thousands of American women can avoid chemotherapy since 43% of diagnosed breast cancer cases fit into the subgroup that is nonresponsive to chemotherapy.

When researchers identify a moderator, they should continue to study separately the different subgroups defined by the moderator. Each subgroup may have a completely different route to the outcome, in which case not separating the subgroups may obscure the answers. For example, research on effective diets for control of obesity has been conducted for years. Still, the "in vogue" diets range from extremely low-fat diets to eat-as-much-fat-as-you-want low-carbohydrate diets, such as the Atkins diet, and no one diet seems to work in the long run. Why do some diets work for some and not for others? And why is there still debate as to which type of diet is best? Perhaps the answers lie in the moderators—that is, some people have a particular reaction to carbohydrates; others, to fats. The challenge of tailoring effective diets perhaps may be met by discovering the moderators of treatment and then by doing the research separately for each type of person.

What Is a Mediator?

In everyday language, a "mediator" is a person who comes between two parties to try to resolve some conflict. Similarly, a mediator in risk estimation comes between the risk factor and the outcome to explain how or why the other risk factor influences the outcome. For example, in Chapter 3, we mentioned that unprotected sex and sharing hypodermic needles are causal risk factors for AIDS. In fact, each of these risk factors is *mediated* by a positive HIV status with respect to AIDS. That is, these risk factors lead to positive HIV status, which in turn leads to AIDS.

> *Mediator: A risk factor that explains how or why another risk factor affects the outcome.*[2,3,9]

A mediator (e.g., a positive HIV status) comes between another risk factor (e.g., sharing hypodermic needles) and the outcome, implying that it "connects" the risk factor to the outcome. However, just as all causal factors are risk factors but not all risk factors are causal, all links in a causal chain leading to an outcome are mediators, but not all mediator chains are causal chains. Since it is so difficult to establish causality, finding mediators points researchers in the right direction. That is, if, for example, excessive alcohol use led to impaired calcium absorption, which in turn led to osteoporosis, then the two risk factors would satisfy the conditions described below in the operational definition for mediation.

Operationally, a risk factor mediates another risk factor for the same outcome, if, in a particular population (1) the two risk factors are correlated, (2) the mediator *occurs after* the other risk factor, and (3) when researchers attempt to use both risk factors to predict the outcome, either both risk factors matter (partial mediation) or only the mediator matters (total mediation).[3]

Consider the rather interesting result described in Example 5.6.

EXAMPLE 5.6

The "News of the Weird" section in *The San Jose Mercury News* (August 24, 2002) states that "researchers at Hebrew Rehabilitation Center in Boston found that the grain in beer (which men consume far more than women) must be a major reason why men suffer less osteoporosis."[10] The newspaper report probably was based on a report in the *American Journal of Clinical Nutrition* exploring dietary silicon intake and bone density. This study found that men had more silicon sources than did women—one of the sources being beer.[11]

If the "News of the Weird" claim of Example 5.6, that beer drinking "must be a major reason why men suffer less osteoporosis," were true, then conceptually beer drinking could be described as a mediator of gender for osteoporosis. This would suggest that beer drinking explains, at least in part, the link between gender and osteoporosis. This still would not mean, however, that this gender-beer link (if it exists) is a causal pathway—this could not be established unless beer drinking was shown to be a causal risk factor—that is, changing the amount of beer people drink affects their risk of osteoporosis.

In our path analogy, a mediator is a bridge between a road (another risk factor) and a destination (the outcome). As illustrated in Figure 5.4, you must cross that bridge to get to the destination. In total mediation, the bridge is the only way to get to the destination; in partial mediation, there are other ways to get to the destination.

Again returning to the example of AIDS infection, unprotected sex and sharing hypodermic needles are probably *totally* mediated by a person's HIV status when AIDS is the outcome. We don't know of people contracting AIDS without first being HIV positive. That is, the HIV infection completely explains why the earlier risk factors led to AIDS. Consider Example 5.7, from Chapter 3.

EXAMPLE 5.7

Phenylketonuria (PKU) is a genetic metabolic disease in which a single enzyme (phenylalanine hydroxylase) is absent. When this enzyme is absent, the essential amino acid phenylalanine builds up in the blood and can cause mental retardation and other neurological problems. Through adherence to a strict diet, children with PKU can expect normal development and a normal life span.

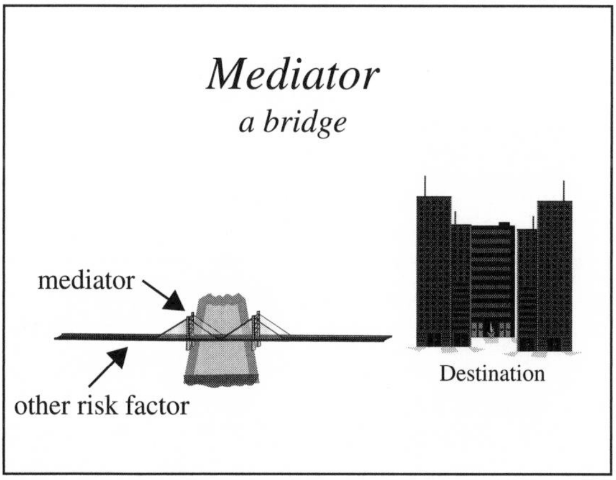

Figure 5.4. An illustrated analogy between a mediator and a bridge.

In Example 5.7, the blood phenylalanine level mediates the PKU gene's effect on mental retardation. That is, the blood phenylalanine level explains why having the PKU gene leads to PKU retardation. In Example 5.4, we discussed another genotype example with respect to childhood abuse and later adult violence. In Example 5.7, however, the genotype moderated another risk factor rather than being mediated by another risk factor. The fundamental difference between these relationships is that, in the PKU example, having the genotype is correlated to the blood phenylalanine level and hence is a mediator relationship. In the example of genetic susceptibility to adult violence, the genotype is not correlated with the abuse,[12] and therefore, the relationship is a moderator relationship.

When a mediator is identified, researchers should attempt to establish whether the path created by the risk factor and its mediator is causal or not. Discovering that the link is indeed causal provides an opportunity to design an intervention to either "knock out the bridge" (if the outcome is undesirable) or "cross the bridge" (if the outcome is desirable).

What Are Independent Risk Factors?

Independent risk factors are essentially the "none of the above" classification to describe the relationship between two risk factors for the same outcome.

Independent risk factors are simply that: independent and unrelated to each other.

> *Independent risk factors: Two risk factors for the same outcome that operate independently from one another—having one risk factor doesn't make it more likely an individual will have the other, and having one risk factor doesn't change how the other might affect the outcome.*

Consider Example 5.8 regarding independent risk factors.

EXAMPLE 5.8

Female gender and being Hispanic American are independent risk factors for obesity.[3] An individual's gender and race are uncorrelated—that is, knowing someone is female does not provide any information about her race, and vice versa, knowing someone's race does not provide any information about his or her gender.

Operationally, researchers identify independent risk factors by not being able to demonstrate that one of the other inter-actions exists. Specifically, independent risk factors are (1) uncorrelated (meaning they cannot be proxy, overlapping, or mediators) and (2) have no time precedence (meaning one cannot be a moderator of the other), or if they do have time precedence, within the subgroups of the preceding risk factor, the potency of the subsequent risk factor is the same (again, meaning the preceding risk factor is not a moderator).

While the courses of action researchers take after identifying one of the other inter-actions involves either setting one aside or somehow considering the pair of risk factors simultaneously, the course of action researchers should take after identifying independent risk factors is to continue to consider and investigate these risk factors separately. This makes sense, because often identifying independent risk factors is really more of a case of being unable to demonstrate one or more of the conditions of the other inter-actions. Thus, this default classification for risk factors encourages work to continue on both risk factors separately until more about each is known.

The gender and race example of Example 5.8 is the simple case of independent risk factors: they are uncorrelated and have no time precedence. Consider a slightly more complex example of independent risk factors when one risk factor does precede the other, described in Example 5.9.

EXAMPLE 5.9

Being born to an HIV-infected mother and receiving blood transfusions during childhood or adulthood are probably independent risk factors for AIDS. Being born to an HIV-infected mother comes before an individual receives (or does not receive) blood transfusions. These two risk factors are probably independent—being born to an HIV-infected mother probably does not make you more likely to receive blood transfusions, and it probably also does not alter the risk of contracting HIV from a blood transfusion. Thus, the relationship of blood transfusions to HIV infection is most likely the same among children of HIV-infected and non–HIV-infected mothers.

In Example 5.9, we are not saying that having two risk factors for AIDS does not make someone more likely to contract AIDS (it probably does!), but, rather, that having the first risk factor does not make the second risk factor more or less likely to produce the outcome. The two risk factors are simply unrelated.

Returning to our path analogy, independent risk factors are simply two different and separate routes to the destination (see Figure 5.5).

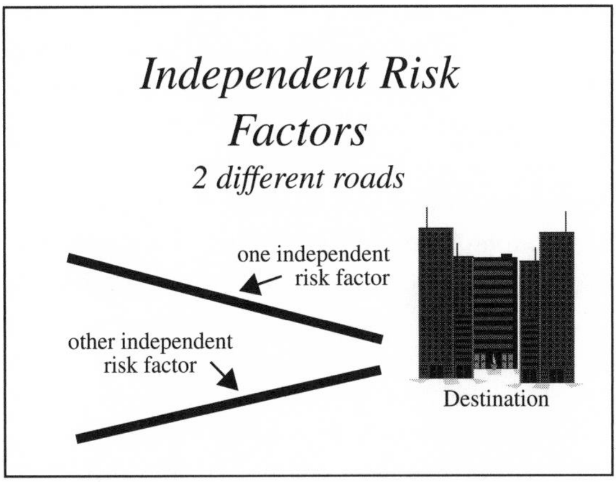

Figure 5.5. An illustrated analogy between independent risk factors and two unconnected roads.

Researchers Use Inter-actions to Sort through a List of Many Risk Factors for the Same Outcome

We have focused here on identifying inter-actions among pairs of risk factors. Nevertheless, if researchers follow a logical order, they can extend this process of pairwise identification to pare down a long list of risk factors for the same outcome. The process itself is like fitting together a jigsaw puzzle. A researcher sorts the pieces (discarding any extraneous ones or duplicated ones) and fits the pieces together two by two until the "picture" or "pictures" emerge. We will step through this process in Chapter 10, but below we briefly list the order of the steps to do this:

1. Sort the multiple risk factors by time.
2. For all the risk factors in each time slot, identify and combine overlapping risk factors and set aside proxy risk factors. This leaves only independent risk factors within a time slot.
3. For all the now remaining risk factors, examine the relationships between earlier risk factors and later ones. If further proxies are found, set these aside.
4. If a moderator is found, split the population on the moderator and begin the analysis anew within each subgroup defined by the moderator.
5. Finally, for all the now remaining risk factors and possibly within moderated subgroups, examine the relationships between earlier risk factors and later ones to identify mediators.

This process is only now beginning to be used in medical research, and, currently, few studies have been published describing such results.[13–15] The experiences we have had to date have been both surprising and encouraging. First of all, when researchers amass the long list of risk factors that have been suggested and/or documented for a particular outcome, they often end up with several hundred. However, when these are all measured in one study (as they must be to follow this process), only a very small fraction prove to be risk factors. Others turn out to be either speculations or nonreplicable results.

Then, a very large number of those risk factors that remain turn out to be proxies or overlapping, further reducing and refining the list. Rarely do researchers find moderators. Usually, finding a moderator is a key finding, but to researchers faced with repeating their analysis within the subgroups defined by the moderator, finding a moderator is not always a joyful event. Then, the mediator chains are often few and relatively simple.

Conclusion and Summary

We present the five inter-actions to illustrate further why we believe a fundamental shift in risk research is necessary. When researchers add yet another risk factor to the pile, often the addition does not increase our understanding of what promotes health and prevents disease, particularly when many of those individual risk factors, by themselves, have very little potency. Our best chance of increasing our understanding and further motivating good research is for researchers to pare down the list to the fundamental core of risk factors, rather than confusing issues by accumulating many different risk factors that ultimately may prove to be the same.

Nevertheless, the true gain in paring down a long list of risk factors by identifying inter-actions is to get to the "meat" of the risk factors: the moderators and mediators. The moderators are instrumental for defining the groups where the results may be different. When these groups are not separated, the results are often blurred. On the other hand, chains of mediators suggest possible causal pathways to be further studied as to whether changing the risk factors in the mediator chains possibly prevents or promotes the outcome. Hence, although we emphasize here the paring down of the list of risk factors by setting aside proxy risk factors and combining overlapping risk factors, we do so to "clear the field" for moderators and mediators. In Chapter 10 we emphasize the value of the moderators and mediators and refer to this paring-down process as "moderator–mediator analysis."

- An "inter-action" describes how two risk factors work together to produce an outcome. Inter-actions allow researchers to "sort out" a list of risk factors to pare it down to its core set and begin to identify causal pathways. We define five inter-actions: proxy, overlapping, independent, moderators, and mediators.
- A risk factor is a proxy to another risk factor for the same outcome if it is only a risk factor for the outcome because of its association with the other, more relevant risk factor. Operationally, a risk factor is proxy to more relevant risk factor if (1) the two risk factors are correlated, (2) neither risk factor precedes the other or the more relevant risk factor precedes the proxy, and (3) when researchers attempt to use both risk factors to predict the outcome, only the more relevant risk factor matters.[3] Proxy risk factors should be set aside.
- Overlapping risk factors are redundant to each other—they either measure the same construct in different ways or they are simply two different names for the same construct. Operationally, risk factors are

overlapping if (1) they are correlated, (2) neither risk factor precedes the other, and (3) when researchers attempt to use both risk factors to predict the outcome, both risk factors matter.[3] Overlapping risk factors should be combined to produce a new, more potent, risk factor.

- A moderator is a risk factor that can be used to divide the population into groups such that within those groups, another risk factor for the same outcome operates differently. Operationally, one risk factor moderates another if (1) the two risk factors are uncorrelated, (2) the moderator precedes the other risk factor, and (3) within the subgroups defined by the moderator, the potency of the other risk factor is different. Often gender is a moderator for many outcomes because frequently the risk factors for a particular outcome are different for men than for women. When a moderator is identified, further research on the outcome should be undertaken separately for the different subgroups.
- A mediator is a risk factor that explains how or why another risk factor works to influence the outcome.[2,3,9] Operationally, a risk factor mediates another risk factor for the same outcome if, in a particular population, (1) the two risk factors are correlated, (2) the mediator occurs after the other risk factor, and (3) when researchers attempt to use both risk factors to predict the outcome, either both risk factors matter (partial mediation) or only the mediator matters (total mediation).[3] When a mediator is identified, further research should attempt to establish whether the path created by the risk factor and its mediator is causal or not.
- Independent risk factors are simply that: independent/unrelated to each other and to each other's effect on the outcome. Operationally, researchers identify independent risk factors by not being able to demonstrate that one of the other inter-actions exists. Specifically, independent risk factors are (1) uncorrelated, and (2) either they have no time precedence or, if they do have time precedence within the subgroups of the preceding risk factor, the potency of the subsequent risk factor is the same. Independent risk factors should be further studied separately.
- A researcher would apply these principles by identifying multiple list factors and using these principles, first to sort the risk factors (removing proxies and combining overlapping risk factors), then fitting the risk factors together two-by-two until the picture emerges of the path to the outcome.

- The "meat" researchers are looking for in this paring down process are the moderators and mediators. Moderators are instrumental for defining the groups where the results may be different. When these groups are not separated, the results are often blurred. Chains of mediators suggest possible causal pathways to be further studied as to whether changing the risk factors in the mediator chains possibly prevents or promotes the outcome. We later refer to this paring down process as "moderator–mediator analysis."

II

How to Recognize Good and Bad Research

Designing a good research study is probably one of the greatest challenges researchers face. Sometimes design decisions are driven by time and budget constraints; other times they are driven by convention and precedence set in that researcher's particular discipline. Either way, Part II is devoted to looking at the advantages and disadvantages of the different ways researchers might conduct studies—specifically, how researchers select participants to be included in a study (sampling, Chapter 6), how researchers conduct the study (research design, Chapter 7), and how researchers measure risk factors and determine whether or not a study participant has the outcome (measurement, Chapter 8).

Although we separate sampling, design, and measurement into three separate chapters, each of these topics is intricately tied to the other two. Researchers do not and cannot make decisions about these topics sequentially or independently. How researchers recruit and select study participants, for example, influences how they can conduct the study. How they conduct the study influences what measurements they can use. What measures they plan to use influences whom they can include in the study. These are all tough decisions that researchers have to make simultaneously, not sequentially as our presentation order of these topics might imply.

Our goal for Part II is to empower the nonresearcher to recognize the benefits of good research as well as the "danger signs" of bad research. For the researcher, we hope to motivate a shift from easier ways of conducting research to ways more likely to produce credible results.

6

Who Was in the Study and Why Does That Matter?

Sampling

> 1936: The *Literary Digest* reports Alf Landon will beat Franklin D. Roosevelt by more than 20% of the vote.
>
> 1948: The *Chicago Daily Tribune's* headline the morning after the presidential election reads: "DEWEY DEFEATS TRUMAN."
>
> 2000: The TV networks announce Al Gore has defeated George W. Bush for the presidency.

All three of these predictions were wrong—very publicly wrong. In 1936, the *Literary Digest* asked 2.3 million voters who they were going to vote for in order to predict that Landon would beat Roosevelt by more than 20% of the vote. Unfortunately, the 2.3 million people the *Literary Digest* asked were magazine subscribers or owners of telephones or cars—a group of people who, indeed, were more likely to vote for Landon, but not a group who represented the nation's voters during the Great Depression.[1]

Sampling errors such as these also arise in risk estimation, but unfortunately, instead of just waiting until after an election to find out we have the wrong (or right) answer, we might wait several years or even decades until conclusions are shown to be erroneous by new research. During this time, many people's lives and well-being may be adversely affected. In this chapter, we describe good sampling practices and caution against other practices likely to result in misleading conclusions.

What Is Sampling?

In Part I we stressed how risk and risk factors can be drastically different in different populations. Recall Example 1.2, in which early research estimated a risk of 80% or more for breast cancer among women with mutations in the *BRCA1* and *BRCA2* genes. The women in the studies that estimated this risk tended to be women who had *both* the mutation *and* a family history of the disease—a different and smaller population than women with only the mutation. Some experts have surmised that the exaggerated risk estimate may have led some women with just the mutations to have their breasts removed.[2]

If researchers could study every member of a population, then sampling errors would not occur. For example, if researchers could study all women, check whether or not they have the mutation, and then watch to see if they develop breast cancer, then the researchers could calculate the exact risk of breast cancer among women with this mutation. Of course, researchers cannot do this. They can only "draw a sample"—that is, recruit a group of women willing to participate in the study and hope that the results drawn from this smaller group generalize to all women.

Unfortunately, even when the sample does appear to appropriately mirror the population of interest, when the gender, age, and other pertinent demographics match those of the population of interest, other sampling errors can still taint the results. For example, in 1996 the three major television networks predicted that Bob Dole would finish third in the Arizona primary. He finished second. Pollsters attributed the mistake to Pat Buchanan supporters who actively sought out and gave their opinions to the pollsters.[1] In other words, not only who the researchers recruit, but how they recruit them can have a significant impact on the results.

In this chapter, we discuss the different ways researchers sample a population. First, we consider several ways of generating a sample likely to produce sound results. Then we consider several other unfortunately common ways of generating samples likely to produce biased and possibly misleading results. Although many of these ways of generating a sample are appropriately used to provide preliminary information necessary for designing a better study, we can also provide many examples when the results of these studies have been used as the basis for medical decision making and have led to poor decisions.

Naturalistic Sampling Is the Most Common Way to Draw a Representative Sample

Suppose a researcher wants to collect a *random sample* of children one to two years of age who currently attend a licensed day care facility in California.

Random sample: A sample drawn from a population such that every member of the population has an equal chance of being included in the sample.

A random sample appears to be the logical first step to study, for example, how the quality of day care relates to future school performance. To collect such a sample, researchers could obtain a list of licensed day care facilities and contact each facility to obtain a list of attendees. They could number each attendee in the appropriate age range and then generate random numbers to randomly select the desired sample size.

In theory, researchers could draw a random sample in this way. But consider the logistic nightmare of obtaining a list of attendees from each day care facility. If researchers were successful at obtaining a list of all attendees, what happens when some of the selected study participants refuse or are unable to participate? Plus, time will elapse between when the researchers obtain the list and contact the chosen participants. During this time, some children will enter day care and some will leave. No matter how hard researchers try, *not* every member of the population of interest will have an equal chance of being included in the sample. Even with the best intentions, this sample will not, strictly speaking, be a random sample.

While random samples are always cited in statistical textbooks, rarely do researchers ever use a true random sample in medical research. Usually, researchers do not have access to everyone in the population of interest (e.g., those in other geographical locations or those not yet born). Moreover, not everyone in the population of interest is likely to agree to participate in a study.

However, the purpose of seeking a random sample is to generate a *representative* sample from the population of interest, that is, a sample in which the distributions of characteristics of interest (e.g., 51% boys, 49% girls) are similar to those of the population of interest.

Representative sample: A sample drawn from a population such that the distributions of the relevant characteristics match those of the population of interest.

For example, to draw a representative sample of children one to two years of age in licensed day care facilities in California, researchers could randomly select several day care facilities and then randomly sample only within the selected facilities. Every child in the population of interest does not have an equal chance of being included. In fact, only those in the selected facilities do. Nevertheless, the selected sample will, ideally, be similar to one drawn randomly from the population, if drawing such a sample randomly were possible.

Naturalistic sampling: A method by which researchers attempt to draw a representative sample. Researchers propose specific inclusion and exclusion criteria, recruit eligible persons, and obtain informed consent.

The most common way to draw such a representative sample is by naturalistic sampling. Even with the best intentions, a naturalistic sample can never be guaranteed to be representative of the population of interest. Anyone considering using the results of a study using naturalistic sampling will typically look at the statistics describing the sociodemographic and relevant clinical characteristics of the sample to determine whether it is "close enough" to the population to whom they hope to apply the findings.

After researchers draw a naturalistic sample, they can look at study participants as they are currently, look at past behaviors, events, and characteristics (study them "retrospectively"), and/or follow the participants for a period of time and look at future behaviors, events, and characteristics (study them "prospectively").

In Prospective Sampling, Researchers Draw a Sample to "Look Forward"

When researchers draw a prospective sample, they intend to follow the participants for some duration of time to observe whether or not the outcome of interest occurs. In Chapter 2 we referred to such a forward-looking study as a "longitudinal" study and in Chapter 7 we discuss further the attributes of longitudinal studies. While in this context "prospective" and "longitudinal" are synonymous, we choose to use the word "prospective" with respect to sampling to clearly differentiate it from its opposite, retrospective sampling.

In our example of sampling children in day care facilities, we described how researchers draw a naturalistic sample and then follow these children prospectively to study future school performance. That is, we described a "prospective naturalistic sample." However, suppose these researchers were, instead, interested in studying risk factors for childhood leukemia rather than future school performance. While virtually all children will have a "future school performance," very few will have childhood leukemia. To be able to generate enough cases of childhood leukemia to study, researchers need an extremely large sample size. For example, if 1% of the population will have an onset of a disorder within the next five years (i.e., an incidence of 1%—probably much higher than the incidence of childhood leukemia), then more than 10,000 participants would have to be studied to be assured of observing 100 onsets of the disorder. Naturalistic samples may run to many thousands of individuals. Such studies are extraordinarily costly in time and money both because of the large sample size and the costs of following each participant over many years. One less costly but viable alternative to naturalistic sampling is *two-stage prospective sampling.*

Two-stage prospective sampling starts off as does naturalistic prospective sampling. Researchers select inclusion/exclusion criteria and implement a sampling method. During the screening procedure, researchers also assess selected risk factors of interest for all participants to be included in the naturalistic sample (stage 1). From this stage 1 information, researchers obtain estimates of the distributions of the selected risk factors in the population (e.g., gender, age). Then, the sample is divided into groups ("stratified") where each group has a particular set of the selected risk factors (e.g., women older than 65, women 65 and younger, men older than 65, men 65 and younger). Researchers then choose a sample size to select from each group ("stratum"). From each stratum, researchers randomly sample the selected sample size and follow only those selected to determine the outcome (stage 2).

> *Two-stage prospective sample: A sample that researchers draw from a population in two stages and follow prospectively. In stage 1, researchers draw a naturalistic sample and collect information on specific risk factors of interest. In stage 2, researchers divide participants into groups ("strata") based upon the risk factors. Researchers then draw a random sample (of size determined by the researcher) from each stratum and follow each for a predetermined duration of time.*

Researchers typically draw a two-stage prospective sample when the outcome of interest is rare and they already know of some risk factors associated with a higher incidence of the outcome of interest. Researchers use known risk factors so that they can carefully select more participants from the strata with a higher risk of the outcome in order to end with more cases of the outcome of interest with a smaller overall sample size.

Consider Example 6.1.

EXAMPLE 6.1

Suppose 10% of the population has a family history of a disease. Those with a family history of the disease have a 30% risk of having the disease, while those without such a family history, have only a 1% risk. Then, the overall risk in the population is 3.9% [(0.10·0.30) + (0.90·0.01)], but more than three-quarters of the cases would be among that small minority with a family history.

With such a rare outcome described in Example 6.1, to obtain a naturalistic prospective sample with, say 100, cases of the disease, researchers would need more than 2,500 participants (100/0.039). To follow more than 2,500 participants over a number of years might more than exhaust the resources available.

Instead, suppose researchers draw a two-stage prospective sample, as illustrated in Figure 6.1. In stage 1, researchers draw a naturalistic sample (the screening sample) and assess family history. From these data, researchers estimate the probability of having a family history of the disease in the population sampled. Researchers then stratify the stage 1 sample into those with and without a family history. Given its rarity, researchers might choose to select all of those with a family history of the disease (10% of the screening sample) and *randomly* select only 11% of those without a family history of the disease to proceed to stage 2. Why 11% of those without a family history of the disease? Researchers can choose any percentage, but a good choice would yield about an equal number of "high-risk" study participants (here, those with a family history of the disease) and "low-risk" study participants (here, those without a family history of the disease). Since researchers chose everyone with a positive family history (10% of the screening sample), they can choose 11% of the 90% without a family history to also equal 10% of the screening sample.

If everyone in stage 1 had been followed up as a naturalistic prospective sample, approximately 3.9% would have the disease, since the risk in the overall population is 3.9%. By drawing a two-stage prospective sample, half of the sample has a 30% risk and half of the sample has a 1% risk, yielding an overall 15.5% risk of the disease in the stage 2 sample. Thus, instead of needing to follow more than 2,500 participants to generate 100 cases of the disease, researchers only need to follow 100/0.155 = 654 participants to see 100 cases of the disease.

Two-stage prospective sampling is an attractive strategy for risk estimation, particularly when the selected risk factors to be used for stratifying in stage 1 are easy for researchers to measure, such as gender, age, ethnicity, geographical location, socioeconomic class, or family history. The analysis of the results, however, is a bit more complex because researchers need to weight the results of stage 2 back to the proportions of each stratum in the stage 1 sample. That is, suppose when researchers conducted the study of Example 6.1, they found that 28% of their stage 1 sample who had a positive

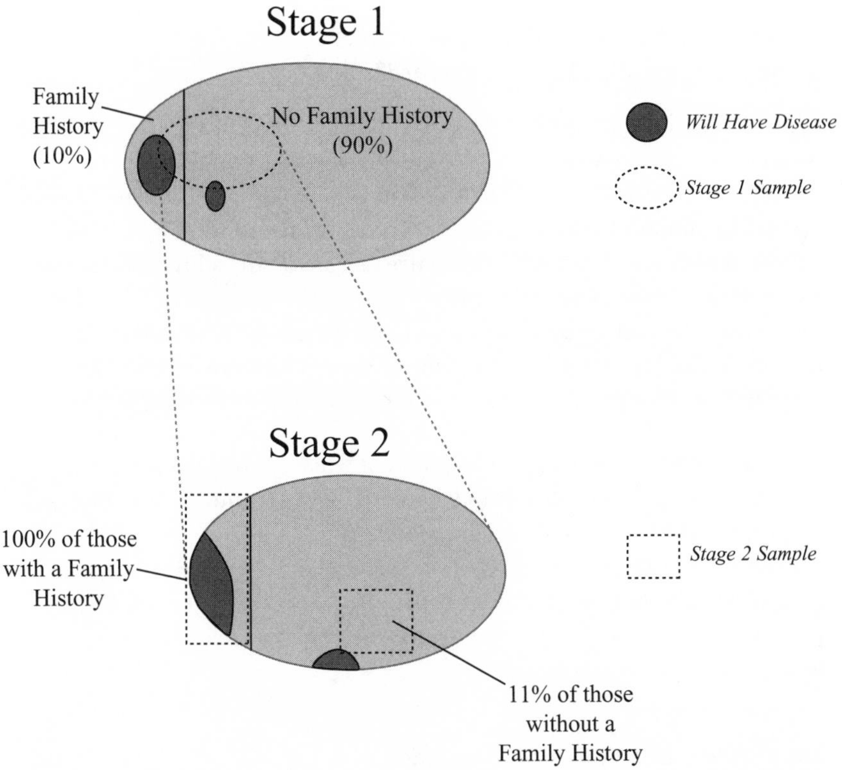

Figure 6.1. An illustration of how researchers might draw a two-stage prospective sample. The left portion of the population (the oval) represents those who have a family history of the disease (10% of the population), while the right portion represents those without a family history (90% of the population). In stage 1, researchers draw a prospective sample depicted by the dotted circle. In stage 2, researchers select 100% of those with a family history (the left dotted rectangle) and 11% of those without a family history (the right dotted rectangle); 50% of the stage 2 sample has a family history and 50% do not.

family history also had the disease (vs. the real 30%), while only 1.2% of those without a family history had the disease (vs. the real 1%), they would then correctly estimate that (0.90·0.012) + (0.10·0.28) = 3.9% of the overall population would have the disease. Any other findings, such as the proportion of those who smoked versus did not smoke, would also have to be weighted accordingly. Methods to apply such sampling weights are well developed,[3] but anyone considering the results of a study using a stratified sampling scheme, such as two-stage prospective sampling, should check that the results are indeed weighted.

In Retrospective Sampling, Researchers Draw a Sample to "Look Backward"

Suppose that instead of following the children prospectively to study some future event, researchers decided to "look backward," sampling children who had already experienced that event or not. For example, suppose researchers wanted to sample children with and without asthma to see if how long each child had been breast-fed was a protective risk factor for asthma. Such a study would be a retrospective study: researchers would use records or retrospective recall to see if the length of time a child is breast-fed is related to whether or not the child has asthma at the time of the study. Studying risk factors in this way has three problems that may lead to questionable results:

1. The population is likely to be different when researchers start at the outcome and look back than when they start at a time before the outcome has occurred and look forward.
2. Retrospective recall is often unreliable and may even be affected by whether or not the outcome occurs.
3. Researchers may not be able to tell whether the potential risk factor precedes the outcome.

The Problem of a Changing Population

When researchers conduct a prospective risk study, the question they are seeking to answer is, for example, "In 20 years, how many more people in a particular population with this potential risk factor will have this outcome than do those who don't have this potential risk factor?" When researchers try to answer this question retrospectively, the people they select to look at may not be the same as the people they would have looked at had they collected a group of people, checked whether or not they had the risk factor, and then followed them for 20 years to see whether or not they had the outcome. People may have moved out of or moved into the population.

People may be missing from the population studied retrospectively because, for example, individuals with the risk factor may have died from some other condition associated with that same risk factor. For example, suppose researchers studied a sample of 60-year-old men to see if their diet and the exercise patterns 20 years ago were associated with current health outcomes such as obesity, high blood pressure, high cholesterol level, or diabetes. The answers they get might be different from the answers they would have had if they had collected a sample of 40-year-old men and followed them prospectively for 20 years. Diet and exercise might also affect whether or not some of these men died between 40 and 60 years of age. Researchers sampling the 60-year-old men would not even know about the men who died before age 60.

Alternatively, people may move into a population if, for example, the community studied has a noted clinic specializing in the particular outcome or if its environment was better suited for managing the condition. For example, a retrospective sample of people with and without asthma from places with little pollution may be very different from a prospective sample of people not yet having had onset of asthma in the same locale. Asthma sufferers from other locales might be attracted to move to low-pollution areas.

The net result is there is no guarantee that a sample collected after the outcome has occurred is representative of the same population to which a researcher intends to apply the findings.

The Problem of Retrospective Recall

Although many potential risk factors of interest may be either fixed markers (e.g., gender or ethnicity) or variable risk factors that were recorded before the onset of the outcome, many factors researchers examine in a retrospective study can only be based on retrospective recall of the participants. "Were you abused as a child 20 or more years ago?" Not only is such recall often unreliable, but it may actually be affected by the experience of the outcome. For example, retrospective recall of child abuse after onset of major depression may be quite different from that obtained from the same person before onset of major depression. In the childhood leukemia example, parents of leukemia patients might recall, for instance, particular chemical exposure their child had only because their child's diagnosis of leukemia influenced them to think long and hard about all past exposures. Parents of children without leukemia probably haven't spent the time painstakingly reviewing their child's life in an attempt to understand why their child might have contracted, but didn't contract, such a disease.

The Chicken-and-Egg Problem: Does the Risk Factor Precede the Outcome?

By definition, a risk factor must precede the outcome. But in retrospective studies, researchers are not always able to tell whether an outcome occurred *after* some potential risk factor was in place. Consider Example 6.2, discussed in Chapters 1 and 2:

EXAMPLE 6.2

In a study described in an article titled "Study Links Sleeping to Attention Problems,"[4] researchers questioned parents about their children's sleep habits, distractibility, forgetfulness, and fidgeting. Researchers found that kids who snored were more likely to also exhibit symptoms of hyperactivity.

Because the study described in Example 6.2 was conducted retrospectively using parental report, there is no way of knowing if the sleep disturbances preceded the attention problems or if the attention problems preceded the sleep disturbances. In addition, this study also has the second problem with retrospective studies: the problems with retrospective recall. As we mentioned before, researchers cannot tell whether the parental reports were accurate or tainted by either the child's sleep disturbances or hyperactivity. That is, parents of children with sleep disturbances may have their own sleep interrupted and be more tired and more likely to view and report their children's daytime habits negatively. Alternatively, parents of hyperactive children may experience more stress, have more disturbed sleep themselves, and then witness and report more sleep disturbances among their children. There are many plausible explanations for the finding—explanations that would not apply had the children been followed prospectively.

Consider a particular type of retrospective sampling that is one of the most common and often one of the most misleading sampling methods in risk estimation: case-control sampling. In case-control sampling, researchers recruit one group of people who have the outcome of interest and another group of people who do not.

> *Case-control sampling: A sampling method in which researchers recruit two groups of people: those with the outcome (the "cases") and those without (the "controls"). Researchers compare various risk factors between the cases and controls to attempt to discover whether some are more prevalent in one group. Researchers often attempt to control the variation between individuals from each group by "matching" controls to cases based on preselected factors of interest (e.g., gender, race, age).*

Consider Example 6.3, a classic example of a case-control study.

EXAMPLE 6.3

In 1981, a study published in the *New England Journal of Medicine* suggested that coffee use might be a cause of pancreatic cancer.[5] The study was a case-control study based on 369 hospitalized patients diagnosed with pancreatic cancer (cases) compared to 644 control patients who had been admitted to the hospital by the same doctor—typically a gastroenterologist. The results were striking—those who drank two cups per day had almost twice the risk than those who did not drink coffee, and those who drank three or more cups per day had almost three times the risk.

At first glance, the results of Example 6.3 seem so convincing that you may even be tempted to skip that second cup of coffee. However, first consider who the controls were. They were largely hospitalized patients of gastroenterologists—doctors who treat diseases and disorders of the digestive system. Many of these patients, either by their own choice or their doctors' orders, were limiting their coffee intake because of their digestive problems. So when these patients were compared to those diagnosed with pancreatic cancer, of course they drank less coffee!

Case-control sampling has all of the possible problems of retrospective sampling we discussed above: the problems of a changing population, retrospective recall, and the inability to determine whether the "risk factor" precedes the outcome.

However, on top of that, case-control sampling has even more salient problems. Since never in the process of drawing a case-control sample do researchers draw a representative sample, the likelihood that the cases and the controls are representative of the cases and noncases in the *same* population is low (a problem known as "Berkson's fallacy").[6–8] Once again, generalizing to a population different from the one that the sample represents can be, and often is, misleading.

The population of hospitalized patients without pancreatic cancer of Example 6.3 is not representative of the general population without pancreatic cancer. Most people in the general population without pancreatic cancer are not hospitalized and are not under the care of a gastroenterologist. And, even if they were, the retrospective nature of this study makes understanding the temporal relationship between coffee drinking and disease state (whether pancreatic cancer or another disease) impossible to sort out.

The problem with the coffee-drinking-and-pancreatic-cancer study was easy to identify. But even when there is no obvious sampling bias, neither we nor the researchers can be sure that other unknown and unknowable factors differentiate the populations from which the samples are drawn and to which the results will be generalized. Consider Example 6.4, from Chapter 4:

EXAMPLE 6.4

A *New York Times* headline claims "Study finds no link between breast cancer and the pill."[9] Scientists at the Centers for Disease Control and Prevention and the National Institutes of Health surveyed 4,575 women who had breast cancer and 4,682 women who did not. They found that 77% of the cancer patients and 79% of the cancer-free women had taken some type of oral contraceptive, suggesting that taking the pill is not associated with a higher risk of contracting breast cancer.

The study described in Example 6.4 was a case-control study, raising concerns about its conclusions. For example, women with a family history or other risk factors for breast cancer may have been discouraged from taking oral contraceptives in the first place, explaining why fewer of the cancer patients ever took oral contraceptives. Researchers did analyze this study from many different angles, such as separately analyzing those with a family history and those without, and still did not find a difference in oral contraceptive use between the two groups. Nevertheless, because of its design, no one can be sure that no other factors differentiate the populations. For example, the cases and controls had statistically significant differences in the number of term pregnancies, family history, and age of menopause[10]—all factors also implicated as risk factors for breast cancer.

Why, then, if the results of case-control studies are so questionable, is this type of study so common in the risk research literature? First of all, case-control sampling is inexpensive and easy to do. The results are often dramatic and easily publishable. Also, case-control sampling is well established by tradition.

A case-control study is justifiable as a preliminary exercise to a better designed risk study. The concept is logical: why not compare those with a disorder and those without to see what the differences may be? In such a study, researchers get experience with diagnosis and measurement of possible risk factors, with dealing with participants in the population of interest, and some "ballpark" ideas as to whether certain risk factors are worth pursuing and how. All such information, when used as a pilot study to prepare for a more definitive risk study, may save much time, effort, and financial investment in that future study. From this point of view, case-control studies are not meant to communicate to decision makers, but to communicate with other scientists contemplating further research.

Unfortunately, many researchers do not consider case-control studies only as pilot studies. Because this methodology is so ingrained in some disciplines and so well established by precedence, researchers conduct many case-control studies to "answer" questions that could only be answered by more difficult and more expensive ways of collecting samples and conducting studies.

There are two additional problems related to sampling worth mentioning that may produce incorrect or misleading answers. One problem arises when researchers sample more than one population and then combine the samples. The other arises when researchers sample people appropriately, but then study "person-years" instead of persons.

Researchers Must Carefully Present the Results of Multisite Studies

Researchers have developed many different sampling strategies to generate large enough samples to study a particular outcome well. Yet even with these different strategies, researchers may still not generate enough cases of the outcome in one geographical area for a successful study. Even when researchers can find enough cases, the population represented is limited to that geographical area. To deal with both these problems, researchers often conduct one study in multiple locations—that is, they conduct a "multisite study." Researchers' intentions are to pool the data from all the sites to generate one set of conclusions.

In a multisite study, each site has its own research staff that follows exactly the same research protocol, including the same sampling protocol. Even when researchers do follow the exact same protocol, however, each population will be geographically different and often sociodemographically and clinically different as well. Results may differ from site to site. However, since all the sites follow the same research protocol, such differences are likely to reflect true population differences and provide either assurance or doubt as to whether the results are generalizable to populations other than the ones selected.

Conducting multisite studies has many advantages. One disadvantage, however, becomes apparent when researchers simply ignore the fact that they are conducting studies with more than one population using different research staff. They often "muddle" the data, that is, throw all the data together and then analyze the data as if they came from one site only. Instead, researchers should "pool" the results by examining the results at each site, comparing the results across sites, and combining the results (not the raw data) appropriately. To see why this is so, consider Example 6.5, which describes a hypothetical example of a two-site study.

EXAMPLE 6.5

Suppose researchers study whether being male is a risk factor for some hypothetical illness. Figure 6.2 illustrates hypothetical results for each of two sites.

The conclusion is the same at both sites, and the pooled result is that being male is *not* a risk factor for this disease. However, suppose site 1 and site 2 each sampled the same number of participants and that the data were thrown together, site ignored (i.e., muddled), as shown in Figure 6.3.

The muddled results would indicate that being male *is* a risk factor for the disease, even though there is no site at which this claim has any support. In fact, if we apply our recommended potency measure of number needed to take (NNT), the NNT = 1.6, suggesting that being male is a very potent risk factor for the disease.

The counterintuitive results from the muddling of data described in Example 6.5 are an example of Simpson's paradox.[11–14] In this extreme example, Simpson's paradox occurs because the prevalence of the outcome is different (the prevalence of the disease at site 1 is 90% and at site 2 is 10%),

Site 1

	Male	*Female*	
Sick	81%	9%	90%
Healthy	9%	1%	10%
	90%	10%	

Site 2

	Male	*Female*	
Sick	1%	9%	10%
Healthy	9%	81%	90%
	10%	90%	

Figure 6.2. Hypothetical results for a two-site study investigating whether men are more likely to have a particular disease. At site 1, 90% of the population is male, and 10% is female; 90% of both the men and the women are sick, suggesting no relationship between gender and having the disease. At site 2, 10% of the population is male, and 90% is female; 10% of both the men and the women are sick, also suggesting no relationship between gender and having the disease.

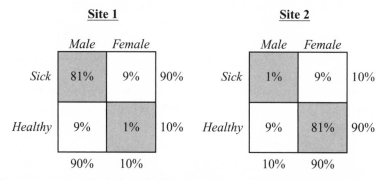

	Male	*Female*	
Sick	41%	9%	50%
Healthy	9%	41%	50%
	50%	50%	

Figure 6.3. Hypothetical "muddled" results for a two-site study investigating whether men are more likely to have a particular disease. Here, 92% of the men have the disease, while only 18% of the women do, suggesting that men have a higher risk of the disease.

even though the association between gender and outcome at the two sites is the same. Simpson's paradox may occur in any situation when the sites differ—either in the associations or in the prevalences. In fact, both sites could have a strong relationship, but the muddled data may indicate no relationship. When samples are drawn from multiple sites, researchers must take site differences into consideration because the muddled results may be completely uninterpretable and misleading. Thus, if a multisite study presented only muddled results, even if each site's study were excellent, the conclusions may be simply wrong.

One argument researchers might make for ignoring site differences, however, is that studies submitted to the Food and Drug Administration (FDA) for the purpose of approving drugs are almost always multisite and almost always muddle the sites. The FDA has provided standards of how to conduct efficacy research. These standards, however, do not require representative samples from populations with the indication for the drug. In fact, several studies have indicated that a large proportion of those who might later use a drug (e.g., sometimes as much as 90%) are excluded from FDA studies.[15] In addition, the FDA requires only statistical significance, not a demonstration of clinical significance. For these reasons, the standards set by the FDA for licensing of drugs are not applicable to risk estimation studies.

Counting Years Instead of People Can Also Produce Misleading Results

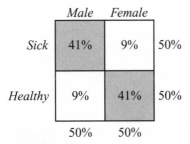

Up to this point, we've discussed different sampling plans in which individual people are sampled. Now we discuss another often used method in which researchers use person-time (e.g., person-years) as the sampling unit. Instead of comparing events per person between a treatment and control group, researchers compare the number of events per person-time. Consider Example 6.6.

EXAMPLE 6.6

In 1985, researchers reported results from the Nurses' Health Study cohort investigating hormone replacement therapy (HRT) as a protective risk factor for coronary heart disease.[16] In this study, researchers used a large naturalistic prospective sample of female registered nurses. There were 32,317 postmenopausal women who, at the beginning of the study, were free of coronary disease. Researchers followed these women for varying lengths of time, resulting in 54,308.7 person-years for women who took HRT ("users") and 51,477.5 person-years for women who did not take HRT ("nonusers"). There were 30 coronary events among users, resulting in an incidence rate of 30/54308.7 = 0.0005524, and 60 events among nonusers, resulting in an incidence rate of 60/51477.5 = 0.001166. Researchers reported what they called the "relative risk" of coronary events as 0.0005524/0.001166 = 0.4738, or about 0.5. Citing this relative risk of 0.5, the researchers concluded that "postmenopausal use of estrogen reduces the risk of severe coronary heart disease."

The study described in Example 6.6 was instrumental in the wide prescription of HRT over the next 15 years, until recent randomized clinical trials began to call these results into question. However, what exactly does a relative risk of 0.5 mean? Calling this number a "relative risk" suggests that HRT users have half the risk of a coronary event than do nonusers. However, we cannot interpret the results this way because the sampling units were person-years, not people.

The rationale for counting multiple years from the same individual as separate entities and pooling these years across individuals stems from a mathematical model called the "constant hazards model." The "hazard" at each point of time is the risk of the event in the subsequent period of time among those who survive to that point of time. A "constant hazard" would mean that the probability of an outcome in the first year of study is the same as the probability in the second year for those who do not have the outcome prior to that time, is the same as the probability in the third year for those who do not have the outcome yet, and so on. Under this assumption, researchers can count three disease-free years from one study participant as three separate entities, exactly the same as one disease-free year from three different study participants. One reward is that the sample sizes become very large: 32,317 women become 105,782.2 woman-years.

However, in the HRT example, it is contrary to empirical evidence to assume that a 30-year-old woman's risk of dying from coronary disease in the next year is the same as a 50-year-old woman's risk. Age itself is a risk factor for death from coronary disease. The hazard among older women (and men) increases each year; it is not constant.

In risk research, the only times a constant hazard model might apply is when the outcome is certain for all people (e.g., death) and when increasing age is not a risk factor. Such examples are hard to come up with—probably only accidental deaths from being hit by a car or lightning would apply. Even being hit by a car might be questionable because older people do not move as fast, do not hear or see as well, and may be more susceptible to being hit by a car than are younger people. The constant hazards model certainly does not apply in the HRT example, since a large proportion of women die free of coronary disease, and among women who survive to an older age, the risk of coronary disease is not constant but increases.

Why, then, did the researchers choose to look at person-years rather than simply persons? At a guess, the reason was that researchers followed each participant for different amounts of time: until she had a coronary event, the study ended, or she dropped out of the study (by, e.g., refusing further participation in the study or death from something other than coronary disease). Counting people in this case is problematic because whether or not a person had the outcome depended on the length of time she was studied—and this length of time was different for different participants. However, there are better ways to deal with studies designed this way. We will refer to these methods collectively as "survival methods."

In survival methods, researchers compare the "survival curves" from those with and without a potential risk factor. Two survival curves are depicted in Figure 6.4: one curve represents the survival among patients who took a drug, and the other curve represents the survival among patients who did not. A survival curve is a plot of the percentage of people in the population who are still outcome-free against time elapsed. Thus, at the beginning of a prospective study (time zero), no one has yet experienced the outcome, so the percentage of people who are outcome-free is 100%. As time progresses and more and more people experience the outcome, this curve drops.

In a prospective study, all survival curves start at 100%, since no one has the outcome at the beginning of the study. Some survival curves end up at zero or 0%, indicating that everyone in the population will, if they live long enough, experience that outcome sooner or later (e.g., menarche or menopause for women, death from all causes in the general population). Other survival curves, like the no-drug curve in Figure 6.4, may eventually stabilize at a proportion or percentage greater than zero, indicating that not everyone will experience that event in their lifetimes (e.g., graduating from college, getting married, having onset of heart disease or Alzheimer's disease). In fact, in the no-drug survival curve, 60% of the population never experiences that outcome.

In risk estimation studies, researchers compute survival curves for those with and without a potential risk factor. Then, if these curves are the same, the factor is not a risk factor. If they are different, the factor is indeed a risk factor. When researchers study participants at a fixed follow-up time (e.g., five years), they are effectively comparing risk at one time point of the survival curve. In comparison, when researchers follow participants for varying

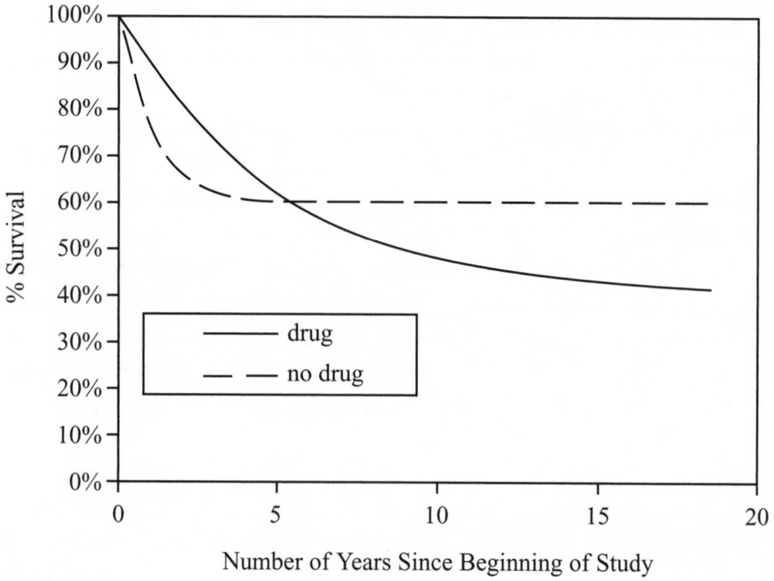

Figure 6.4. A sample survival plot. The vertical (Y) axis represents the percentage of people in each population who are outcome-free. The horizontal (X) axis represents the number of years since the beginning of the study. In the first five years of the study, more people taking the drug (the solid line) are outcome-free than are people not taking the drug (the dashed line). After about five years, the curves cross such that more people who do not take the drug are outcome-free than those taking the drug. After about three years, 60% of the people who did not take the drug remain outcome-free for the duration of the study, while the percentage of people who take the drug who remain outcome-free steadily declines.

lengths of time, they record when the event occurred (if it did). The survival curves generated by these data allow researchers to compare the risks in the groups at any time point up to the total duration of the study. Thus, survival curves contain much more useful information about risk than would any outcome defined at a fixed follow-up time.

In particular, notice how the survival curves in Figure 6.4 cross after about five years have elapsed. Thus, a study that used a fixed follow-up time of three years would say that the survival rate among those taking the drug was better, but another study that used a fixed follow-up time of seven years would have the opposite result!

Consider Example 6.7, in which survival analysis was used to show that psychotherapy was protective against death from breast cancer.

EXAMPLE 6.7

Researchers compared the survival curves of women diagnosed with breast cancer who received usual care (the control group) and those who received usual care plus psychotherapy (the treatment group). Up to about two years of follow-up, the survival rates of the two groups were about the same. However, after that time, the curves started to diverge. Women in the treatment group survived longer than those in the control group, suggesting that psychotherapy in combination with usual care (e.g., chemotherapy and/or radiation) was protective against death from breast cancer in this population.[17]

What is particularly interesting about the study described in Example 6.7 is that researchers detected no difference in survival in the first two years. Had the design of this study been to follow women for one or two years and then determine how many in each group survived, the conclusions would have indicated that psychotherapy makes no difference with regard to survival. The longer the fixed follow-up time, the stronger the protective factor would appear to be.

When using survival methods, researchers record a time for each participant. If the participant has had the outcome, researchers record the time that outcome occurred. If the participant has not had the outcome, researchers record the time at which follow-up for that person was discontinued. Such a discontinuation time is called a "censored survival time," in that it acknowledges that the time of the outcome for that person (if it ever occurs) must be longer than the recorded time. Using this information, researchers can estimate the survival curve using, for example, Kaplan-Meier analyses.[18,19]

However, these methods run into problems when censored times and the survival times are somehow related. Such a relationship exists when the same causal factors affect the timing of the outcome and the likelihood of discontinuation of follow-up. For example, participants could drop out because they died of other diseases that share the same risk factors as the outcome of interest. In the HRT study of Example 6.6, researchers also analyzed the results using a survival analysis model. However, HRT is a known risk factor for certain types of cancer, which may account for many of the noncoronary heart disease deaths (there were 379 total deaths, of which only 90 were due to coronary heart disease). In the analysis with death from coronary heart disease as the outcome, deaths due to other causes were apparently counted as censored survival times—that is, they were counted the same as if the woman had dropped out of the study. Had these women not died first of these other diseases for which HRT is a risk factor, they might have been at greater risk of a coronary event. In other words, these HRT users were counted as contributing "coronary heart disease-free" years, but by virtue of dying of something else (also possibly associated with HRT), they lost their chance of contributing to any incidences of coronary heart disease. Could this problem also explain why the conclusions of this study ultimately proved so questionable?

Conclusion and Summary

In this chapter, we have presented ways to collect a sample likely to produce an unbiased result as well as ways to collect a sample likely to produce a biased, and possibly misleading, result. Many of the sampling methods that we urge not be used as a basis for medical decision making—retrospective sampling, case-control sampling, use of incidence rates—are quite common in risk research primarily because they are easier ways to get an answer quickly. In many cases, these quick answers are exactly what researchers need to design better risk studies for future research. Unfortunately, all too often these quick "answers" hit the press and are interpreted as the true answers before additional research is conducted or even considered—as in the 15 years between the initial HRT studies and the Women's Health Initiative study on HRT. The fundamental shift in risk research we are urging is a shift from these easier, but also often misleading, ways of collecting a sample to the ones more likely to produce credible and reproducible results.

How researchers collect the sample is closely aligned with how they plan to conduct the study. In Chapter 7 we discuss the different ways researchers conduct studies and what appropriate conclusions can be drawn from each.

Many of the issues that arise in research design are mirrored in sampling—typically the quickest and easiest ways to conduct a study are also the ways most likely to be overinterpreted and produce misleading results.

- Researchers cannot typically study every member of a population (e.g., all U.S. women over the age of 65). Instead, researchers must "draw a sample," that is, study some of the people from the population of interest in hope that the results drawn from this smaller group are generalizable to the entire population of interest.
- Even when the population studied appears appropriate, the method by which researchers draw the sample can lead to misleading or erroneous conclusions.
- A random sample is a sample drawn from a population such that every member of the population has an equal chance of being included in the sample. Although often cited in statistical textbooks, true random samples are almost never used in medical research since, for several reasons (e.g., some people are not available or not willing or able to participate), it is almost impossible to include every member of a population with equal probability.
- A representative sample is a sample drawn from a population such that the distributions of relevant characteristics match those of the population of interest.
- Naturalistic sampling is a method by which researchers attempt to draw a representative sample. Researchers propose specific inclusion and exclusion criteria, recruit eligible persons, and obtain informed consent.
- A two-stage prospective sample is a sample researchers draw from a population in two stages and follow prospectively. In stage 1, researchers draw a naturalistic sample and collect information on specific risk factors of interest. In stage 2, researchers divide participants into groups ("strata") based upon the risk factors. Researchers then draw a random sample (of size determined by the researcher) from each stratum and follow each for a predetermined duration of time. The advantage of this sampling scheme is that it allows the researcher to sample more people from the higher risk strata so that they can observe more cases of the outcome with a smaller sample size.
- In retrospective sampling, researchers draw a sample to "look backward." Retrospective sampling is problematic because (1) the population is likely to be different when researchers start at the outcome and look back compared with when they start at a time before the out-

come has occurred and look forward, (2) retrospective recall is often unreliable, and (3) it is difficult to tell whether the potential risk factor precedes the outcome or the outcome precedes the potential risk factor.

- Case-control sampling is one type of retrospective sampling in which researchers recruit two groups of people: one group with the outcome (the "cases") and another group without (the "controls"). Researchers compare various risk factors between the cases and controls to attempt to discover whether some are more prevalent in one group. Case-control studies share all of the problems of retrospective studies. In addition, it is never clear that the cases and controls represent the cases and controls in the same population. Although case-control studies are valuable as pilot studies to better designed, prospective studies, the results of case-control studies should not be used as the basis for medical decision making.
- A multisite study is one study conducted at multiple sites. Each site is geographically distant from each other and has its own research staff that each follows exactly the same research protocol for sampling, measurement, and design. Researchers pool the data from all the sites generating one set of conclusions. Misleading results can occur from multisite studies if researchers "muddle" the data, that is, treat the data as if they came from a single site, rather than analyzing the results separately at each site and then pooling the results appropriately.
- Looking at incidence rates, such as the number of events per people-years, is typically inappropriate because the assumptions required to analyze data in this way (the constant hazards model) are seldom valid in risk research.
- We strongly advocate use of survival methods as long as there is no relationship between if and when a participant drops out of the study (the "censored time") and if and when the outcome occurs. When such a relationship exists, for example, when the same risk factor leads to death from the outcome of interest and death from other causes, the results may be misleading.

7

What Is the Difference between a Risk Factor and a Cause?

Research Design

Could certain animal species potentially warn us of impending earthquakes? In the late 1970s, Stanford researchers attempted to answer this question by observing whether they could detect behavioral changes in chimpanzees prior to earthquakes. Many local farmers and animal lovers shared their convictions with the researchers that their livestock or pets behaved strangely before earthquakes. One dairy farmer was particularly insistent that his cows "acted up" before an earthquake. When researchers urged him to call as soon as he witnessed such behavior, he responded indignantly he couldn't: "Until I know there was an earthquake, how can I know why the cows were acting up?"

The challenge of risk estimation is to recognize the signs of an impending event *before* the event happens. Only what happens before an event gives clues as to the causes of that event. Only before the event happens can we hope to intervene to prevent the event. That risk factors be shown to precede the outcome is thus the most vital part of the definition of a risk factor and crucial to risk estimation.

In Chapter 6, we stressed that studies based on retrospective sampling or incidence rates (i.e., sampling person-years rather than people) may provide useful information to other researchers doing further research on the topic but should not be the basis of medical decision making. Even if we only consider studies that sample prospectively, we still must be aware of a study's design and maybe, most important, of the study's duration. Can researchers establish time precedence when the duration of study is so short that neither the outcome nor the potential risk factors change between the time the study begins and ends (i.e., a cross-sectional study)? Or must researchers follow participants over a longer duration of time to observe change in the outcome and/or potential risk factors (i.e., a longitudinal study)? These questions speak to the quantity and quality of information that researchers can collect from participants, but equally crucially, they also speak to the cost and the feasibility of the study.

In preceding chapters, we touched upon some merits and problems of cross-sectional and longitudinal study designs. In this chapter, we expand these discussions with the goal of emphasizing that studies that cannot conclusively establish the time precedence of risk factors are of limited value for medical decision making. Moreover, among those studies that do establish time precedence, only a small fraction can support a claim of causality.

Cross-Sectional Studies Are Valuable as Pilot Studies, but Also Have the Potential to Mislead

In preceding chapters, we presented examples of results from cross-sectional studies. Let's discuss in more depth the cross-sectional nature of a result we discussed in Chapter 3: the higher divorce rate among those who live together prior to marriage, as described in Example 7.1.

EXAMPLE 7.1

A report prepared by the Center for Disease Control's National Center for Health Statistics provides many interesting statistics concerning patterns of marriage, divorce, and cohabitation based on data from the National Survey of Family Growth (NSFG) consisting of interviews with 10,847 women between the ages of 15 and 44.[1] For example, 43% of first marriages break up by 15 years. This statistic varies by race (Asians have the lowest rate of divorce), religious affiliation (those with no affiliation have a higher rate of divorce), age of the bride (brides younger than 18 were more likely to divorce than brides older than 25), education, income, and many other characteristics. This report also includes the often-cited result that the rate of divorce is higher among those who lived together prior to marriage than among those who did not live together prior to marriage (51% vs. 39% by 15 years).

Since researchers conducted interviews with participating women once and collected information either about the woman's current characteristics or her retrospective recall, the design of the study described in Example 7.1 was cross-sectional.

> *Cross-sectional study: A study that examines the relationship between potential risk factors and outcomes in a span of time so short that neither the potential risk factors nor the outcomes are likely to change during the duration of the study.*

The cross-sectional design of this study was simple: researchers interviewed each participant once. Researchers did not track participants or interview them repeatedly. Such a design eases the burden both on the participants and on the research staff. Such a design makes it easier to recruit a representative sample of participants from the population of interest because potential participants are much more likely to agree to be interviewed once rather than to return multiple times. Finally, such a design means a much cheaper study, which eases the problem of attracting sufficient funding. Because researchers can generate many publications within a short period of time, such studies are also more career enhancing.

So, if these studies are cheaper and easier, produce more results, are more career enhancing, and, finally, are easier to get funded, why aren't all studies cross-sectional? When the research goal is to identify correlates, a cross-sectional design is adequate and because of its advantages, usually recommended. In fact, when the research goal is only to identify fixed markers (e.g., gender or race), a cross-sectional design is also usually adequate. However, when researchers are trying to identify risk factors that are not fixed, particularly risk factors that could provide the basis of interventions to prevent or promote the outcome, cross-sectional studies are usually *not* adequate. In such cases, cross-sectional studies cannot establish the precedence of the potential risk factors to the outcome. Thus, any identified correlates cannot be established as risk factors, and, if so interpreted, can be misleading. Since our primary interest is identifying risk factors, and, more important, causal risk factors, cross-sectional studies have limited value.

For example, many cross-sectional studies report an association between homelessness and mental health problems. Does poor mental health lead to homelessness? Does homelessness lead to poor mental health? Or perhaps neither leads to the other but some other causal risk factor leads to both? As another example, in the NSFG (Example 7.1), women who had ever had a generalized anxiety disorder had a higher rate of divorce than those had not had such a disorder. But how can researchers tell if the anxiety disorder preceded the divorce or the divorce preceded the anxiety disorder? Cross-sectional studies can only demonstrate that homelessness and poor mental health, or divorce and anxiety, tend to occur in the same people at the same time. Such studies do nothing to establish which, if any, precedes the other.

Cross-sectional studies are a necessary and valuable precursor to designing another type of study in which researchers can establish temporal precedence. The problem arises, however, when researchers or the media proclaim the results of a cross-sectional study in such a way that others are misled. Consider Example 7.2.

EXAMPLE 7.2

In July 1998, researchers reported on an examination of 59 previous cross-sectional studies, concluding that childhood sexual abuse is minimally associated with psychological harm.[2]

The result described in Example 7.2 was highly controversial and ultimately denounced in the U.S. Congress. The study had numerous scientific flaws; for example, the researchers based their conclusions upon a sample of college students (children seriously affected by childhood sexual abuse are less likely to be found in college), and they defined sexual abuse very generally (ranging from witnessing indecent exposure to repeated rape). The cross-sectional design meant the "risk factors" in question (past sexual abuse) were based on retrospective recall—recall that may (or may not) have been affected by whether poor psychological outcomes occurred. If the conclusions were not so obviously politically incorrect and, for that matter, contrary to the results of previous studies, this study, like many other cross-sectional studies with retrospective reports, might have been taken seriously and accepted as "truth." Surely this "truth" could be twisted to exonerate, for example, Catholic priests for sexual abuse of children because "the damage wasn't so bad."

We have already pointed out the problems with retrospective recall—most crucially, recall may be affected by whether or not the outcome occurred. Probably some outcomes are more likely to "taint" the recall than others, but researchers cannot predict which outcomes are more damaging to recall than others. Multiple studies have compared careful recordings to recall and have typically found that recall is poor. Consider Example 7.3.

EXAMPLE 7.3

Danish researchers asked women near the end of their second trimester of pregnancy about recent flu symptoms. After delivery, researchers asked these same women again about the flu symptoms they experienced in their second trimester.[3] Fifty percent of women who reported a fever around 25 weeks of gestation did not recall that fever later at delivery. Likewise, 85% of women who reported a persistent cough near 25 weeks also did not recall that cough at delivery.

The Danish researchers described in Example 7.3 were interested in studying the recall of infections because of a 1958 study that found no relationship between influenza infections during the second trimester of pregnancy and incidence of schizophrenia among the children of those pregnancies. The finding of no relationship contradicted multiple other studies that had supported the link between influenza infections during gestation and future schizophrenia. The Danish researchers hypothesized that the reason this one study had a different result was because it used retrospective recall rather than medical records. Their result suggests that studies based on retrospective recall may get different answers than those based on medical records or some other method of recording events as they happen.

What if the researchers conducting the studies on past sexual abuse had not used retrospective recall but had checked police and/or medical records? Since these records would have been created at the time of the incidents, the events they record would have unequivocally preceded the psychological outcomes measured in college. Of course, a large proportion of sexual abuses may go unreported to either police or medical professionals. Nevertheless, we would be more likely to accept the result *for the population studied* if based on police or medical records, but, as in the reporting of infection during pregnancy example, the result would not likely have been the same.

Using records to establish risk factors is one way in which researchers can establish precedence in a cross-sectional study, since information on the potential risk factors were "collected" (i.e., recorded) much earlier than the outcome measures. Similarly, in a cross-sectional study, researchers can always clearly establish precedence for fixed markers at birth (e.g., gender, ethnicity or race, genotype, year of birth, socioeconomic status of the family at birth, birth weight, birth complications, birth order). In addition, certain factors may become fixed early in life (number of years of education by age 30, age of menarche by age 20, age of first pregnancy by menopause, etc.). Then, a cross-sectional study seeking risk factors for an outcome that happens in later life (postmenopausal breast cancer or Alzheimer's disease) could establish precedence for such risk factors. Of course, the most commonly acknowledged and verified risk factors are fixed markers—these factors are easy to measure. However, while fixed markers are useful for identification of those at high enough risk to warrant intervention, and valuable as clues to possible causal risk factors, they cannot, themselves, be causal risk factors.

As we mentioned in Chapter 1, another often misleading result from cross-sectional studies arises from the use of "lifetime prevalence." Recall *prevalence* is the proportion of a population who have the outcome sometime within the time period of the observation, while *incidence* is the proportion of a population who have *onset* of the outcome within the time period of the observation. "Lifetime prevalence" is a term that refers to the percentage of people in a cross-sectional study who answer "yes" to the question: "Have you ever had this disease?" When researchers ask this question of a population of participants all of the same age, lifetime prevalence is not, in fact, a prevalence at all, but the incidence between birth and that fixed age. Thus, when all participants are the same age, there is no problem except for the peculiarity that an incidence is labeled prevalence. However, typically, when researchers use lifetime prevalence, their study includes participants of different ages. In these cases, the lifetime prevalence is an uninterpretable number completely dependent on the ages of the participants in the sample. Consider hypothetical Example 7.4.

EXAMPLE 7.4

Suppose researchers compute the lifetime prevalence of an event such as menarche (age of first period). If they take a sample of eight-year-old girls, the lifetime prevalence is near 0%. If they take a sample of eighteen-year-old women, the lifetime prevalence is near 100%. If, however, they study different samples consisting of girls of mixed ages between eight and eighteen, the lifetime prevalence depends entirely upon whether the group predominantly includes older girls (in which case the lifetime prevalence would be high) or younger girls (in which case the lifetime prevalence would be low).

But even for outcomes other than menarche described in Example 7.4, many of which become more or less common as we age, the distribution of ages in the sample matters more to the estimated prevalence than does the outcome itself. Generally, a lifetime prevalence can range anywhere between 0% and the percentage of people in the population who, before they die, experience onset. Not surprisingly, different studies of lifetime prevalence of the same outcome in the same population often report wildly different figures for lifetime prevalence.

When lifetime prevalences are used for *both* a potential risk factor and an outcome, the result is likely to be misleading. Consider Example 7.5.

EXAMPLE 7.5

Suppose the potential "risk factor" is whether or not a girl has ever studied geometry, and the outcome is whether or not she has had menarche. If all the participants in a sample are twelve, researchers probably would find no relationship between these two factors: the twelve-year-olds who have studied geometry are probably not more or less likely to have had their first menstrual period, or vice versa. However, if the participants in the sample vary in age, it would probably look like those who have studied geometry are more likely to have had menarche. Those who are youngest in the sample are more likely neither to have studied geometry nor to have had their first period, while the older participants in the sample are more likely to have done both. Such a result might lead some to suggest studying geometry as a risk factor for menarche or, worse, suggest that studying geometry may be a cause of menarche.

For an example such as menarche and studying geometry (Example 7.5), the dependence on the ages of the participants in the sample may seem obvious and trivial, but with other potential risk factors and outcomes such as "Have you ever been in a car accident?" and "Do you have osteoporosis?" the dependence on age may not be so obvious. Unless a study is stratified by age (i.e., the sample is divided into age groups and findings are reported by those age groups), lifetime prevalence used either descriptively or in any analyses can be misleading.

In summary, cross-sectional studies can produce a wealth of information about correlates. Once such correlates are identified, researchers must conduct further studies to establish whether or not these correlates are indeed risk factors. Cross-sectional studies can only establish precedence for fixed factors or factors that become fixed early relative to the outcome. Such studies cannot document causal risk factors under the best of circumstances. Thus, cross-sectional studies are valuable as pilot studies for other longitudinal studies, but they also have the potential to mislead as errors of interpretation are very common—especially when researchers use lifetime prevalences or retrospective recall.

Longitudinal Studies Are the Major Source of Credible Information about Risk Factors

If a cross-sectional design is not adequate to identify most risk factors, what is the alternative? It is a longitudinal design: a more complex and expensive design in which researchers follow study participants over a period of time. Longitudinal studies are the major source of credible information about risk factors, and particularly of the types of risk factors (variable risk factors) that have some chance of being identified as causal risk factors.

> *Longitudinal risk study: A risk estimation study in which researchers collect information from participants over a period of time. At the beginning of the study, all participants are outcome-free. During the follow-up period, researchers repeatedly assess potential risk factors as well as assess whether or not the outcome has occurred.*

Many of the results we have already presented are based on longitudinal studies: "Study links gene to violence in boys who have been abused" (Example 3.6—participants were followed from birth for 26 years); the drug cholestyramine reduces cardiac events by 19% (Example 4.2—participants with high cholesterol were given cholestyramine or a placebo and followed for an average of 7.4 years); the Nurses' Health Study in which researchers concluded use of hormone replacement therapy *reduces* the risk of severe coronary heart disease (Example 6.6—the 32,317 postmenopausal women who were followed for varying numbers of years); and, finally, the more recent and contrary example we discussed in the introductory chapter concerning the Women's Health Initiative's randomized clinical trial (RCT) that was shut down because women on hormone replacement therapy were having *more* heart attacks and strokes than those taking placebos.

Consider perhaps one of the longest-running longitudinal risk studies, described in Example 7.6.

EXAMPLE 7.6

In 1921, Lewis Terman studied 1,528 California "gifted" schoolchildren (IQs exceeding 140). Researchers followed and evaluated these participants in terms of physical and psychological health, as well as in terms of avocations, scholastic achievement, and life accomplishments. Terman died in 1956, and by 2002 many of the children had also died, but the study continues, projected to be completed in 2010 when presumably the last of the gifted children of the Terman study will be deceased.[4] In general, Terman showed that being a gifted child is protective against physical defects and abnormal conditions. Adults who were gifted children were better adjusted mentally and socially than are nongifted children. By age 35, 80% were in the highest socioeconomic groups, compared to 14% of the general population.[5]

Most longitudinal studies are not as long lasting as the Terman study described in Example 7.6, nor, given funding exigencies, can they be. Determining the length of time researchers follow study participants and how often researchers assess participants is one of the greatest challenges in designing a good longitudinal study. Stanford professor Lincoln Moses once suggested that the best way for researchers to plan a research study was to envision how they would prove their point if they miraculously had access to everything they might want to know for every person in the intended population. If they can't do that, needless to say, they certainly can't make their point with the more limited information they can reasonably expect to get! But if they can envision their strategy under the best of circumstances, the trick is to determine the minimum amount of data necessary to accomplish the same purpose. If researchers cannot follow participants from birth to death (and they usually cannot), what is the latest they can start and the earliest they can stop to get the necessary information? If researchers cannot have hourly or daily information about each participant (and they usually cannot), how infrequently can they assess the participants and still make the point? If researchers cannot know everything about each participant, what essential information is enough and how best can researchers measure it?

Fortunately, medical decision makers do not have to make the tough choices with respect to study design—they have only to assess when the study is done whether the researchers have proved their point. But to make that judgment, anyone acting as a medical decision maker needs to have some insight into how researchers' design decisions affect the credibility of the results. When reviewing the results of a longitudinal study, we need to consider the following crucial questions:

- When did participants enter the study, and how many of those screened were ineligible because they had already experienced the outcome? This number should be quite low, certainly less that 25% (i.e., the researchers have to have started early enough to capture most of the cases in the population of interest).
- How many of those who entered the study subsequently had the outcome? This number should be high, at least of the order of 50. That may not seem a stringent requirement, but when the incidence during the follow-up period is, say, 1%, that means a total sample size of more than 5,000.
- What proportion of those entered into the study dropped out? This proportion should be near 0%, although few studies actually achieve 0%. If many drop out of the study, there may be serious biases in the results.

- Did the researchers pay attention to issues such as retention and missing data in their analyses? Loss to follow-up and missing data are inevitable in longitudinal studies. If the researchers do not discuss how they dealt with these problems in the analysis, readers should be somewhat more suspicious of the conclusions.
- As always, did researchers achieve statistically significant results? If the answer is "no," then probably the sample, in one way or another, was inadequate to the task, and the results should be set aside. If the answer is "yes," then how large was the effect, that is, the potency? Was it large enough to be of clinical significance?

In the hierarchy of studies, clearly longitudinal studies are much more valuable to risk estimation than are cross-sectional studies. But even so, as the questions above indicate, much still can go wrong in the design of a longitudinal study. In addition, longitudinal studies can still share the problem of retrospective recall with cross-sectional studies: even a study that reevaluates a participant yearly may have to rely on retrospective recall of events in the previous year. Anyone considering using the results of a longitudinal study still has to carefully examine its methods. Moreover, although a well-designed longitudinal study can provide the crucial information on precedence necessary to establish a risk factor, longitudinal studies that consist of simply observing risk factors and outcomes (i.e., "observational studies") do not provide much, if any, convincing evidence of causality. Studies in which researchers manipulate risk factors to see if such manipulation changes the risk of the outcome (i.e., "experimental studies") provide the most convincing evidence of causality. Figure 7.1 depicts a hierarchy of studies showing how cross-sectional studies form the foundation but are lower in the hierarchy in terms of the information they can provide than longitudinal studies.

As shown in Figure 7.1, cross-sectional studies are always observational. Longitudinal studies, on the other hand, may be observational or experimental. We have already described many observational longitudinal studies: the Terman study of gifted children (Example 7.6), the Nurses' Health Study in which researchers concluded use of hormone replacement therapy reduces the risk of severe coronary heart disease (Example 6.6), and "Study Links Gene to Violence in Boys Who Have Been Abused" (Example 3.6). Consider also Example 7.7.

EXAMPLE 7.7

In the late 1960s, newspapers reported a number of observational studies that suggested that use of analgesics and anesthetics during labor and delivery caused subsequent impairment in the infant.

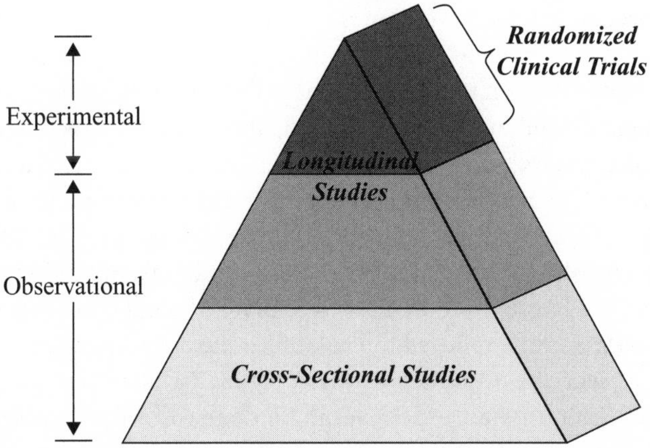

Figure 7.1. A hierarchy of the different types of risk estimation studies. Cross-sectional studies form the foundation of the hierarchy. Studies farther up the hierarchy typically are more difficult and more expensive but also typically produce more information usable to medical decision makers. The pinnacle of the hierarchy is a randomized clinical trial (RCT)—an experimental longitudinal study—probably the most expensive and most difficult of studies but also the one that can provide the most convincing evidence of causality.

The studies looking at the issue of drug use during delivery were longitudinal studies, but they were observational. Further studies indicated that the drugs used during labor and delivery did not lead to the impaired functioning of the infants, but rather the complications and difficulty of the delivery led to a higher likelihood that the mother would use analgesics and anesthetics during labor and delivery and later have an infant with impaired functioning.[6]

While longitudinal observational studies can provide the crucial information on precedence necessary to establish most risk factors, they usually cannot provide convincing evidence of *causal* risk factors. For that purpose, experimental studies, more specifically referred to as RCTs, are the "gold standard."

Randomized Clinical Trials Are as Close as Researchers Can Come to Establishing Causality in a Single Study

Most people consider RCTs as studies to test the effectiveness of an intervention, not studies to check whether a risk factor is causal. In fact, testing the effectiveness of an intervention *is* checking whether a risk factor is causal. When researchers provide an intervention to a treatment group and do not provide an intervention to a control group, they are using an intervention to change something about the study participants in the treatment group with the goal of changing some outcome. When, for example, researchers give participants in the treatment group a drug and give participants in the control group a placebo, they are checking whether taking the drug changes the risk of the outcome of interest. In the cholestyramine example (Example 4.2), researchers used an RCT to demonstrate that reducing cholesterol level by taking cholestyramine reduced the risk of having a cardiac event.

In the hierarchy of studies shown in Figure 7.1, RCTs are the pinnacle. They are difficult, they are expensive, and if done correctly, they can provide convincing evidence of whether a risk factor is causal or not. However, even if we do not consider the costs, sometimes ethics preclude researchers from conducting an RCT. For example, researchers cannot assign some people to smoke in order to establish that smoking causes lung cancer or assign some unmarried couples to live together and others to live separately in order to establish that premarital cohabitation increases the likelihood of divorce.

Ethics can also present challenges when based on previous, possibly misleading, evidence. As we described in Example 7.7, observational studies suggested that drug use during labor and delivery might be associated with the impairment of the infant. With that suggestion, investigators in the early 1970s proposing to do RCTs to test the causal effect of such drugs on infants met resistance from those who approve and fund research protocols. In this way, conclusions based on observational studies may prevent the necessary research from being done. Luckily, researchers found other ways to tackle this issue and without an RCT were able to show the complications during delivery led to a higher risk of impaired functioning, not the taking of pain-relieving drugs. Many mothers-to-be (including two authors of this book) breathed a sigh of relief!

Luckily for medical decision makers, once again their burden is not to figure out the ethical issues that led to the research design, but rather to ascertain the ramifications of the results of a study already designed and conducted. Thus, here we discuss the key components of good RCTs. We do not, however, discuss specific technical design issues because there are many available references on this subject.[7,8]

The goal of an RCT is to show that a risk factor is causal for an outcome. To do this, researchers propose an intervention or treatment designed to change that risk factor—either by removing a risk factor implicated in causing an outcome or introducing a protective factor implicated in preventing that outcome. The treatment may be administration of a drug, psychotherapy, educational program, diet or exercise program, or any strategy that somehow changes the risk factor. Then, to satisfy the definition of a causal risk factor, the researcher must show that the treatment actually changes the risk of the outcome.

Unfortunately, demonstrating that a change in the risk of the outcome is attributable to the treatment is no easy feat. As we have mentioned before, often other factors, such as the characteristics of those who choose a course of treatment or even subconscious biases of the researchers in how they evaluate those who are treated versus those who are not may result in a change in the risk of the outcome among the treated group. Thus, a true RCT has three specific safeguards intended to prevent extraneous factors from influencing the outcome. When these safeguards are in place, any changes in the risk of the outcome are more convincingly attributable to the treatment than to some other unknown factor.

> *Randomized clinical trial (RCT): An experimental longitudinal study having the following three characteristics: (1) the trial includes both a treatment and a control group; (2) researchers randomly assign study participants to the treatment or control group; and (3) the participants and research staff are both "blinded" such that, as much as possible, neither the participants nor the research staff know who is in the control group and who is in the treatment group.*

Each of the criteria for an RCT is discussed in more detail below.

An RCT Includes Both a Treatment and a Control Group

If a risk factor is causal, we would expect a difference in the risk of the outcome between people exposed to the risk factor and those who are not. However, the only way to see such a difference is by studying what happens to those not exposed to the risk factor. In the cholestyramine example, 7.0% of study participants taking the cholesterol-reducing drug cholestyramine had a cardiac event by the end of the study. This statistic is meaningless until it is compared to the 8.6% of study participants taking a placebo who had a cardiac event.

Defining an appropriate control group is always a source of argument among researchers. For example, when researchers recruit participants with the promise of a treatment that might prevent some unpleasant outcome, there may be a "placebo effect." Since recruitment often focuses on "high-risk" individuals, in the period immediately following initiation of treatment (no matter how ineffectual the treatment) all participants may improve simply because they were initially in such a bad state that, crudely put, they couldn't get any worse. Moreover, some apparent improvement might simply result from expectation effects. Finally, simply paying attention to particular study participants can result in an improvement in their condition. For this reason, a comparison group that is initially as similar as possible to the treatment group is necessary. Changes seen in each group cannot be attributed to the treatment, only differences between the two groups.

In drug studies, the control group will often take a look-alike placebo. However, administering a placebo when other effective treatments are available raises ethical issues since it means that known effective treatment is withheld from the control group for the duration of the study. More recently, more drug studies use "treatment as usual" (whatever physicians ordinarily use) or "standard care" (the best choice of currently available treatment) as a comparison to the treatment being studied.

Nondrug RCTs follow similar principles in selecting an appropriate control, although the issues are quite different. For example, in Example 3.7 we introduced the Infant Health and Development Program (IHDP), an eight-site study of low-birth-weight premature infants. In this study, researchers attempted to show that certain environmental conditions were causal risk factors for low IQ among low-birth-weight premature infants. In the RCT portion of this study, families in the control group received "standard care," while families in the treatment group received parental education and support and the children received high-quality day care in addition to standard care.

Researchers Randomly Assign Study Participants to the Treatment or to the Control Group

The best way to understand how exposure to a risk factor affects a particular outcome is to study what happens to individuals when they are exposed to a risk factor compared to what happens when they are not. Unfortunately, researchers cannot observe an individual both exposed to and not exposed to a risk factor at the same time. Even if individuals could, for example, receive the treatment for a period of time and then receive the control condition for a period of time (referred to as a "crossover" design), they still might have changed from the earlier time to the later or might have aftereffects of having taken the treatment given earlier. Thus, crossover designs can produce misleading results.

The only way to compare treatment against control without encountering possible crossover effects is to study one group that undergoes treatment with another group that undergoes the control condition and compare the *average* effects on the outcome within each group. However, in observational studies often both known and unknown characteristics of the individual determine which group they belong to. In such studies, researchers can never be sure that the comparison between the treatment and control groups reflects the effect of treatment rather than of characteristics that relate to the selection of the treatment.

For example, researchers conducting an observational study comparing the number of heart attacks among people with high cholesterol who take a cholesterol-reducing drug to those who do not may find that those with the highest cholesterol levels are the same ones who take the drug. Or, alternatively, those more affluent or having prescription drug coverage and better access to medical care may be the ones who take the drug. All of these factors are alternative explanations for any differences seen between those taking the drug and those not in an observational study. For example, those more affluent or having better access to medical care may have fewer heart attacks. If these same people are the ones who also choose to take the drug, it may look like the drug, rather than the better access to health care, is reducing the risk of heart attacks.

For this reason, *random* assignment of study participants to the treatment or control group is essential for an RCT. Only then can researchers be sure that no selection factor determined who ended in one group and who ended in the other. With random assignment, the two groups are as similar as two different random samples from the same population can be. Of course, by virtue of chance, differences may exist between the groups. For example, when researchers compare the baseline characteristics of the two groups (e.g., age, gender, height, or weight), they should expect 5% of the independent characteristics to be significantly different at the 5% level. In fact, if researchers report *no* differences between the two groups on many baseline characteristics, we would be wise to question the findings. Differences will exist by sheer chance alone.

Everyone who is randomized must be considered in the comparison ("analysis by intention to treat"). If researchers excluded some, for example, because they died or dropped out of the study, sometimes their death or dropout is related to their group assignment. Then, excluding these dropouts could introduce an additional factor that might explain a difference in the two groups. For example, suppose the cholesterol-reducing drug intended to prevent heart attacks actually causes death from other causes. If study participants who die of other causes are excluded from the analysis, it might appear that the drug prevents heart attack deaths because those who dropped out might have been at highest risk of subsequent heart attack deaths as well. Worse yet, the drug may actually increase the risk, a fact that may be covered up by removing the dropouts from the study. In the case of dropouts, often a treatment's effectiveness is tied to how well patients comply. If participants who respond most poorly do not comply or drop out of the study and these are simply eliminated from the analysis, the results may suggest a completely noneffective treatment is effective. Thus, every RCT should be analyzed initially by intention to treat, although secondary analysis might investigate the phenomena of compliance and dropout and attempt to estimate what would have happened if neither had occurred.

Nevertheless, sometimes, for whatever reason, researchers could not or did not randomize. Typically, researchers will use analytic procedures to "control" for this or that factor (sometimes called a "confounder"). However, they can never be sure that they controlled for all the factors, particularly unknown ones that may influence the outcome. In addition, as we said in Chapter 3, mathematically "controlling" for a factor is a matter of applying a particular statistical model. Thus, the results are correct only if the assumptions underlying the statistical model are correct.

The Participants and the Research Staff Should Be "Blinded" to Treatment Group Membership

Often the term "blinded" refers to ensuring that neither the participants nor the research staff know which participants are in the treatment group and which are in control group. However, we here use the term "blinded" a little more generously to mean that researchers take some precautions to ensure that the group assignment does not influence the evaluation of whether the outcome occurs or not. When researchers do not take such precautions, the evaluation could be biased by the opinions of the research staff or their hope that, for example, a treatment will prove effective. Research staff members who interact with the participants could, if they knew who was who, inadvertently convey their beliefs about the efficacy of the treatment to the study participants and/or to those who evaluate treatment, changing expectations or influencing compliance, ultimately influencing the outcome.

In the IHDP example, both the research staff and the participants in the treatment group, of course, knew they were receiving parental education and support and high-quality day care for their children, and the control group knew they were not. However, the IHDP outcome assessors were not part of the research staff at each site. They were contracted to the coordinating center to do the primary outcome assessments blinded to the group membership of the participants. They had no contact with either those delivering the treatment or control interventions.

In summary, RCTs are those based on these three criteria: definition of appropriate control and treatment groups, randomization, and "blinding."

Conducting such a study is as close as researchers can come to documenting that a risk factor causes a certain outcome (or a treatment prevents or cures it) and, by far, the easiest way. In evaluating whether the evidence is convincing that risk factor is causal, everyone should examine the report for these three key concepts: control, randomization, and blinding. If any of them are missing, anyone intending to use the results should be a little more careful about accepting the conclusions.

Conclusion and Summary

The path of least resistance in risk estimation studies is a cross-sectional study: simple, inexpensive, fast, and easy to publish. However, this path is very limited in its yield of results likely to elucidate the causes, prevention, or cures of medical outcomes. A harder path is longitudinal studies, which are difficult, costly, and time-consuming, but the only path to the most valuable risk estimation results for medical decision making. However, such studies still cannot establish causal risk factors. Finally, the hardest path is a special type of longitudinal study, the RCT, the only path that can provide convincing evidence of causality of a risk factor for an outcome. This type of study is particularly important to decision making in that it documents what interventions might prevent or promote outcomes. While an RCT is expensive and time-consuming, in the end it may not be more expensive or more time-consuming than the multiple and different studies required to provide convincing evidence of causality without an RCT. Worse yet, an RCT is also probably not more expensive and time-consuming (and probably less dangerous) than taking action based on results from other studies that were easy, but possibly wrong.

Just as how researchers sample study participants is closely tied to how they are going to conduct the study, how researchers both sample and conduct the study is also closely tied to what measurements they can use. Even the best study designs may not produce great (or even any) results if researchers cannot accurately measure the potential risk factors or outcomes of interest. Thus, Chapter 8, the last chapter in this section on recognizing good and bad research, focuses on how measurement quality affects research results.

- A cross-sectional study is a study that examines the relationship between potential risk factors and outcomes in a span of time so short that neither the potential risk factors nor the outcomes are likely to change during the duration of the study. Such studies consist of, for example, a single interview, examination, or survey administered once.

- Cross-sectional studies can establish precedence only for those potential risk factors that are fixed markers or factors that become fixed prior to the time the outcome is expected (e.g., age of first pregnancy for an outcome typically occurring after menopause). For other factors, cross-sectional studies can only show that the factor and outcome are correlates, not risk factors.
- A longitudinal risk study is a risk estimation study in which researchers collect information from participants over a period of time. At the beginning of the study, all participants are outcome-free. During the follow-up period, researchers repeatedly assess potential risk factors as well as assess whether or not the outcome has occurred.
- The design of a longitudinal study must strike a tricky balance between being long enough to observe enough occurrences of the outcome and being short enough to not lose or lose track of participants (or even research staff). The study must begin tracking participants at a young enough age and follow them for a long enough time to observe most of the possible occurrences of the outcome.
- An observational study is a study in which researchers simply observe what happens to participants: researchers estimate the risk of a particular outcome among participants with one or more particular risk factors by comparing how many participants with and without the potential risk factor experience the outcome. Observational studies cannot establish causality, because those with the risk factor may also have other known or unknown characteristics that influence the outcome.
- An experimental study is a study in which researchers manipulate one or more potential risk factors for some of the participants (the treatment group) and not others (the control group) and compare how many participants in each group experience the outcome.
- A randomized clinical trial (RCT) is an experimental longitudinal study that includes a control/comparison group, randomizes participants to the control or treatment groups, and "blinds" the assessment of outcome to group membership by whatever means necessary. RCTs, if done correctly, provide the most convincing evidence of causality for a risk factor.

8

What Else Should We Pay Attention To?

Reliability and Validity of Measurements and Diagnoses

You see a doctor for a strange pain in your foot. The doctor says you have a rare disease that will eventually lead to disability unless you have surgery that will render you unable to walk for at least six months. What should you do? Most people would answer: "Get a second opinion!" Why? Because a diagnosis is not a disease. A diagnosis is a doctor's educated opinion of what may be going on, but it may not be correct. In this case, you hope it's not.

In the same way, a measurement of some characteristic is not the entire characteristic, but one view of what that characteristic is. You go into a physician's office and have your blood pressure taken by the nurse. A few minutes later, the physician might also take your blood pressure and find it to be different. After a few minutes' rest, the physician might take it again and find it to be different yet again. A single blood pressure measurement does not completely determine a patient's "true" blood pressure, since blood pressure varies from minute to minute, depending on the circumstances. For example, some people may be more anxious—and thus may experience a rise in blood pressure—when the doctor is present. Moreover, the doctor and the nurse may place the cuff differently, inflate the cuff differently, and even read the outcome differently.

In Chapters 6 and 7 we described good and not-so-good practices with respect to sampling and study design. We are already seeing the shift in risk research from some of the ways that are more likely to produce misleading results to the ways we recommend of conducting research. However, one more key element to ensuring that research reaches, as much as possible, the "right" answers is often overlooked: measurement. That is, how well researchers measure the risk factors and the outcomes of interest has a major impact on the results. Diagnoses and measuring blood pressure are simple illustrations of how measuring an outcome or a risk factor is usually not straightforward.

Measuring a risk factor imprecisely is like trying to watch a movie through dirty glasses or glasses with the wrong prescription—the dirtier the glasses or the worse the prescription, the less likely you will be able to see the movie. Measuring an outcome imprecisely is like watching an old or poorly projected movie—the worse the projection, also the less likely you will be able to see the movie. When you have both a problem with your glasses and the movie's projections, you are probably not going to see the movie at all. When risk factors are measured poorly and/or when outcomes are measured poorly, researchers have a very difficult time seeing exactly what's going on. They may have a negative result—that is, they may not find a statistically significant association between the hypothesized risk factors and the outcome—when really what's happening is that the tools they are using to see the risk factors and/or the outcome are too imprecise to see the associations that really exist.

The terms "validity" and "reliability" describe measurement quality. In this chapter, we define these terms and discuss the impact poor validity and poor reliability have on research results, how researchers assess validity and reliability, and what strategies researchers use to improve measurement quality.

What Are Validity and Reliability?

Measurement quality describes how well a measurement matches the true "thing" researchers are trying to measure. If researchers, for example, want to measure cognitive ability using an IQ score, the measurement quality of the IQ score describes how well an IQ score measures cognitive ability. In casual conversation, people often use the words "validity" and "reliability" interchangeably to mean how good the measurement is. Nevertheless, validity and reliability are actually two different concepts quantifying two different sources of variability in measurement. Consider Example 8.1.

EXAMPLE 8.1

An article titled "Study Reveals Problems in Measuring Kids' Heights"[1] described a study in which staff at primary care practices received extra training in how to measure kids' heights. Before the training, researchers found that only 30% of measurements were within one-half of a centimeter of a measurement taken by a experienced pediatric endocrine nurse using "correct technique and equipment."[2]

The study described in Example 8.1 looked at height measurements of 878 children. Of course, the height measurements varied from child to child. This variation is attributable to three sources:

1. The different heights of the children
2. Other things specific to each individual child (e.g., how straight the child stood, or how much the child moved during measurement)
3. Random error in the measurement not specific to the individual child (e.g., the nurse wrote down the wrong number, or the equipment was misaligned)

In something as ostensibly simple as measuring a child's height, we would expect most of the variation in child's height to be attributable to the first source—children receive different height measurements because they are different heights. The study in Example 8.1 showed, however, that not all the variation can be attributed to how tall the child actually is (what we will call "the relevant information"). If all the variation could be attributed to the relevant information, then the trained nurse using the correct technique and equipment should have gotten the exact same number as the doctor or nurse who originally measured the child in the primary care physician's office.

The other two sources of variability—other things specific to each individual child that influenced their height measurement (or "irrelevant information") and random error—also affected the number recorded as that child's height. These three sources of variability are depicted in Figure 8.1. As this figure shows, validity describes how much of the variability is attributable to relevant information; reliability describes how much of the variability is attributable to relevant *and* irrelevant information or, equivalently, how much of the variation is *not* attributable to random error. Random error is simply that—error that occurs on a random basis and is not specific to a particular child, such as a nurse misrecording a measurement, or the measurement equipment getting misaligned or malfunctioning in some way. A reliable measure will be relatively impervious to these random variations that may or may not occur during one particular measurement. Thus, regardless of what "random stuff" occurs during each measurement, a reliable measure will yield similar results when repeated.

> *Validity of a measurement/diagnosis: The proportion of the variability of a measurement or diagnosis that can be attributed to relevant information in a specified population, that is, how well in a specified population the measure or diagnosis represents the characteristic or disorder of interest.*

> *Reliability of a measurement/diagnosis: The proportion of the variability of a measurement or diagnosis that is not due or random error or, alternatively, how well researchers can reproduce a measurement or diagnosis on repeated trials in a specified population.*

An easy way to think about and remember reliability and validity is to consider the disease or characteristic to be measured as a target. One measurement or one diagnosis is one dart being thrown at that target, as depicted in Figure 8.2. The reliability of that measurement or diagnosis is represented by how well multiple darts thrown at the target for the same

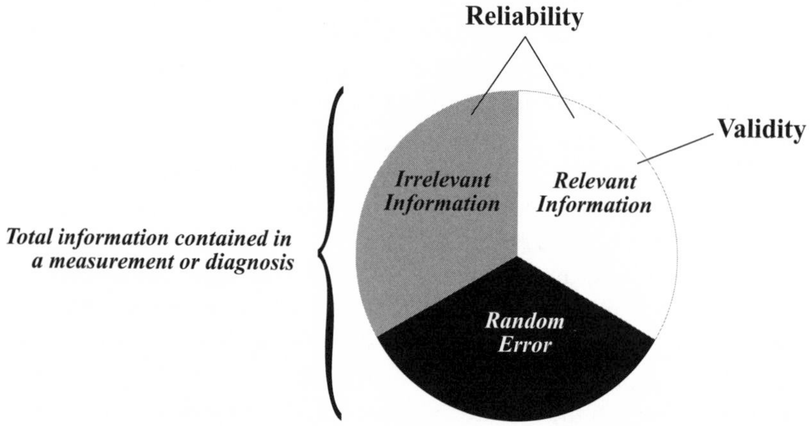

Figure 8.1. A breakdown of the total information contained in a measurement or diagnosis. Reliability measures both the relevant and irrelevant information, reflecting how little random error exists. Validity measures only the relevant information, that is, how well the measurement measures the characteristic.

individual end up in the same place. The validity is represented by how close to the bull's-eye each dart gets, where the bull's-eye is what researchers intended to measure.

If we move the target but keep throwing the darts the same way, the reliability remains the same—the darts may hit a different spot on the target, but how close the multiple darts thrown for the same individual are to one another is the same. As we see in Figure 8.3, however, the validity changes as the location of the bull's-eye moves. Thus, reliability describes a measure (a dart), while validity involves consideration of both a measure and the characteristic or disorder of interest (the dart and the target).

For example, when researchers use an IQ score to measure cognitive ability, validity describes how well an IQ score measures cognitive ability while reliability measures how well repeated IQ tests yield the same score for the same person. If instead of cognitive ability, however, researchers choose to use an IQ score to measure predicted school performance, the validity of an IQ score changes, but the reliability does not. Thus, the proportion of relevant versus irrelevant information conveyed by the measure changes depending on the characteristic or disorder of interest, but the total of those (i.e., the reliability) does not.

Over the years, there has been a good deal of discussion and dissension about the validity of an IQ score as a measure of cognitive ability, but there has been little dissension that an IQ score is a reliable measure. An individual's IQ score typically does not change too radically from one sitting to another. However, the validity of the IQ score when measuring cognitive ability has been called into question. Other characteristics of an individual, completely

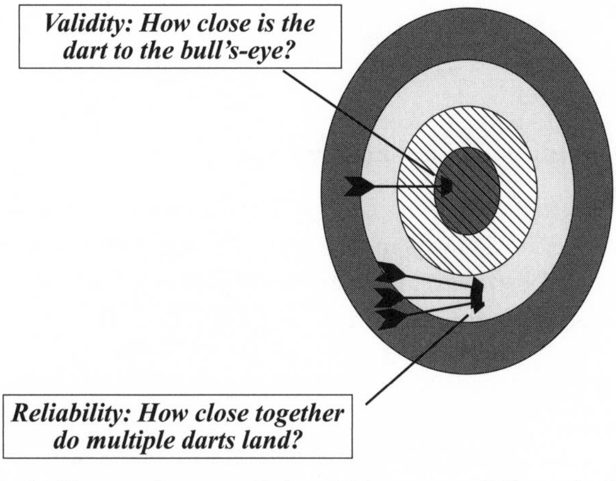

Validity: How close is the dart to the bull's-eye?
Reliability: How close together do multiple darts land?

Figure 8.2. An illustrated way to distinguish between validity and reliability.

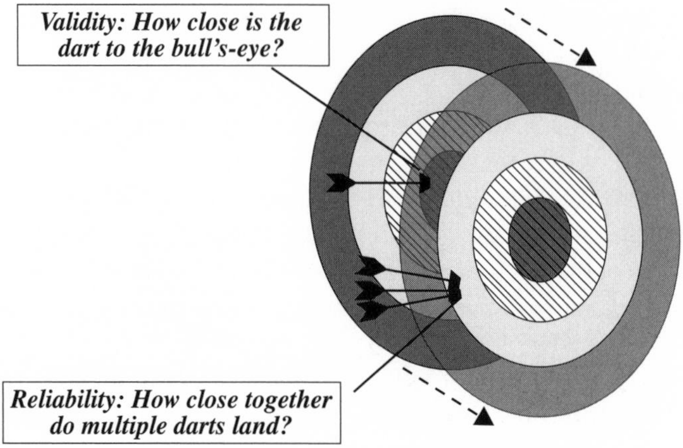

Figure 8.3. How validity and reliability change when the intended target changes. Moving the target changes how close the darts are to the bull's-eye (validity) but not how closely each strike the same spot (reliability).

separate from cognitive ability, also influence his or her score, such as a child's primary language, cultural background, and strengths and weaknesses in areas of competence not measured. In other words, even if an IQ score were perfectly reliable (i.e., the darts hit the target in the same place every time), the score is not necessarily valid (i.e., the darts may be hitting six inches to the left of the bull's-eye).

Validity is part of reliability. A measure that is perfectly valid must be perfectly reliable, because a perfectly valid measure has no random error. Or in other words, if the darts all hit the bull's-eye (valid), they are all landing in the same spot (reliable). However, as the example above about IQ score illustrates, a measure can be perfectly reliable but not necessarily valid.

Why Are Validity and Reliability Important?

In the introduction of this chapter we used the analogy of trying to watch a poorly projected movie through dirty glasses to illustrate how poor measurement quality can obscure results. Example 8.2 provides a more concrete medical example of how poor measurement quality can obscure results.

EXAMPLE 8.2

Suppose researchers could calculate a "breast cancer score" for 35-year-old women based on genetics, family history, health indicators, and so on. Suppose that those who will develop breast cancer within the next 20 years score much higher than those who will not develop breast cancer in the next 20 years. Suppose 20 years ago researchers measured this score completely reliably and validly for a group of 35-year-old women and now know who developed breast cancer. Line (a) in Figure 8.4 depicts a hypothetical set of scores for those who have breast cancer (the black dots) and those who do not (the white dots). Such a result would be terrific if this clear delineation between those who will have breast cancer and those who will not held true with a much larger sample size. Then physicians could foretell who will get breast cancer and take appropriate action.

Now suppose the breast cancer scores were not perfectly reliable, but rather that there was some random error in the scores. Then the

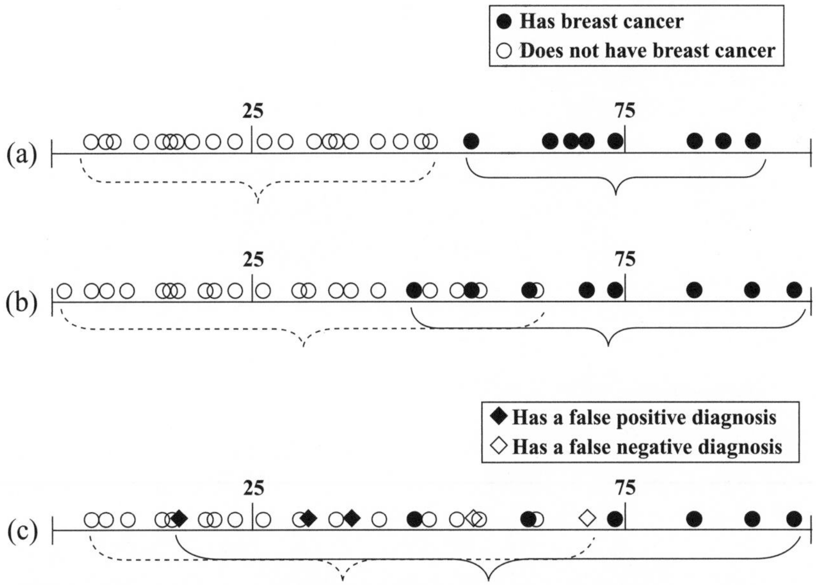

Figure 8.4. An illustration of why poor measurement quality in the risk factor or the outcome can obscure results. Lines (a), (b), and (c) show different scores for a hypothetical breast cancer metric measured 20 years ago. On line (a), none of the scores of individuals who have had breast cancer in the last 20 years (the black dots) are lower than the scores of those have not had breast cancer (the white dots). In line (b), we introduce error in the scores, such that the some of the scores of individuals who had breast cancer overlap with the scores of individuals who did not, making the score a less valid and less reliable predictor of breast cancer. In line (c), we introduce error in the diagnoses of breast cancer such there is little differentiation in scores between those who have had breast cancer and those who do not.

pattern of dots might look more like line (b) in Figure 8.4. The average score in the high-risk and low-risk groups remains the same (about 25 in the low-risk group, 75 in the high-risk group), but the unreliability spreads out or "blurs" the measures in the two groups. Now the overlap in the two groups means a physician would be no longer able to completely accurately foretell who might get breast cancer.

Finally, suppose in addition to the unreliability of the scores, some of those diagnosed with breast cancer were incorrectly diagnosed ("false positives"), and some who were not diagnosed actually had breast cancer ("false negatives"). Then, as depicted line (c) of Figure 8.4, the overlap between the high- and low-risk groups is even greater, perhaps to the extent that distinguishing the two groups becomes impossible.

In Example 8.2, the consequence of low reliability of either the measurement or the diagnosis is a loss of differentiation between the low- and high-risk groups. In risk research, this would also correspond to a loss of potency of a risk factor. When the potency is attenuated, the sample size necessary to detect any nonrandom association becomes much larger. Results are likely to prove "not statistically significant." Even when they are statistically significant, the potency might suggest trivial importance.

The consequence of low validity is even more obvious to comprehend, but maybe not as easy to illustrate. Simply put, if researchers are not measuring what they claim to be measuring, then decisions can be misled. Consider Example 8.3.

EXAMPLE 8.3

A current debate regarding the risk benefit ratio of treating children and adolescents with a class of antidepressants (selective serotonin reuptake inhibitors, or SSRIs) has been fueled by suggestions that SSRIs may increase (not decrease) the risk of suicide in children with depression. British authorities have limited the use of SSRIs in children and adolescents unless prescribed by specialists. In the United States, the Food and Drug Administration recommended a review of all data (published and unpublished) relating to the use of SSRIs in children and adolescents. One such review study has suggested that children who take SSRIs have almost twice the risk of suicidal tendencies (3.2% vs. 1.7%). Since no child in any of the studies reviewed actually committed suicide, researchers focused on suicidal behavior and thoughts to describe "suicidality." However, critics argue that many of the "suicide-related" events were inaccurately classified. Proponents of the study argue that even if inaccuracies occurred, they should have affected both the drug and placebo groups such that the final answer would be the same. Critics counter with the argument "garbage in, garbage out"—those who take the drug, for example, might have more energy and are more likely to have events misclassified as suicidal.[3]

Example 8.3 highlights the importance of measurement because ultimately the entire issue of whether a class of drugs might be removed from the market for use in children may come down to how reliably researchers measure suicidality, and then how valid is a measure of suicidality when the outcome of interest is suicide.

How Do Researchers Assess Validity and Reliability?

The first thing to keep in mind before considering how researchers assess validity and reliability is that reliability and validity describe a measurement or a diagnosis in a particular population. So, for example, the reliability and validity of measuring an adult's temperature using an oral thermometer are probably high. On the other hand, the reliability and validity of measuring a very young child's temperature this way may be quite low since most young children are unable to keep the thermometer under their tongue for the requisite amount of time.

Assessing reliability of a particular measure or diagnosis is much easier than assessing validity, primarily because reliability is not dependent on what is intended to be measured or diagnosed. For this reason, many more studies assess reliability than assess validity. And for this reason, we first discuss how researchers assess reliability.

Assessing Reliability

Assessing reliability of a measurement or diagnosis in a population simply requires checking how well multiple measurements (taken independently of one another) of the same individual match. Typically, researchers will use a correlation coefficient as an estimate of the percentage of total information conveyed in the measure that is free from random errors: a "reliability coefficient."

Researchers speak of different types of reliability: test–retest reliability, interobserver reliability, intraobserver reliability, and so forth. Test–retest reliability refers to how similar repeated testings yield the same result (e.g., if someone takes two IQ tests a week apart, how similar are the two scores?).

Interobserver reliability describes how similar are the results from two different "judges" (e.g., how similar are two blood pressure readings—one taken by a nurse, the other by a doctor?). Intraobserver reliability describes how similar are the results from the same "judge" measuring twice (e.g., if a pathologist reviews two tissue samples from the same patient—assuming he or she doesn't recognize that the samples are the same—how well do the two diagnoses match?). Which type of reliability is appropriate depends on what sources of errors researchers anticipate to be most important. If the measurement is subjective (as in a diagnosis), then a major source of error is likely who is making the diagnosis, in which case interobserver reliability may be most important. On the other hand, with an objective test, such as an IQ test, who administers the test probably does not matter as much as does the inconsistency of the individual's response from one time to another in the relevant span of time. Then test–retest reliability may be most important.

While there are no absolute standards of what constitutes "good" reliability, typically test–retest reliability coefficients greater than 0.8 are considered "almost perfect," 0.6–0.8 "substantial," 0.4–0.6 "moderate," 0.2–0.4 "low," and below 0.2 "inadequate."[4] However, these guidelines may shift some depending on the outcome and the population. A reliability coefficient greater than 0.8 means that more than 80% of the variability among individuals is due to either relevant or irrelevant information specific to the individual and *not* due to random error. Less than 0.2 means that more than 80% of the variability is due to random error. Consider Example 8.4.

EXAMPLE 8.4

The "best" measure of obesity has been in debate for many years. Researchers have used several measures ranging from body mass index (BMI) to measures that estimate the body's fat composition (e.g., skin-fold measurements, bioelectrical impedance, hydrostatic weighing, imaging technologies). A researcher might check the reliability of one such measure by having different testers measure each individual and calculating the correlation between the measurements (interobserver reliability). One such study estimated the reliability of bioelectrical impedance, skin-fold fat, and hydrostatic methods by having each participant tested four times by two testers on two different days. They found all three methods to have reliability coefficients ranging from 0.957 to 0.987—all quite reliable.[5]

While the different measures are considered reliable in Example 8.4, in Example 8.5 the reliability is more questionable.

EXAMPLE 8.5

Eight different expert pathologists rated a set of 37 skin tumor samples as benign, malignant, or indeterminate. The estimated interobserver reliability coefficient (kappa) was 0.50, indicating moderate agreement among the eight experts. However, in only 13 of the 37 cases (eight benign/five malignant) did the eight experts unanimously agree. The samples used for this study were submitted by the same experts who rated the samples. These experts chose these samples for their "classic features." The authors suggest that the reliability of diagnosis of malignant melanoma may even be *worse* for samples not selected for their "classic features" among diagnosticians not selected for their expertise.[6]

Example 8.5 provides yet another illustration of why a second opinion is usually a good idea. With respect to risk estimation, the example also illustrates why the reliability of the outcome measure (typically a diagnosis) is a very important consideration.

Assessing Validity

Although assessing reliability of a measurement or diagnosis is not too difficult, assessing validity is quite difficult and sometimes impossible. To assess how well a measure or diagnosis represents the characteristic or disorder of interest, researchers need something to measure that characteristic or disorder of interest (a "gold standard") with which to compare the measure of interest. This presents a "catch-22" situation: if researchers had a gold standard in the first place, they may not even care about how well another measure measures the characteristic or disorder of interest. Researchers wanting to establish that, for example, an IQ test is a valid measure of cognitive ability need some sort of standard that unequivocally represents cognitive ability. If they had such a standard, perhaps they would not need an IQ test.

On the other hand, the gold standard, if it exists, is not always more desirable than another measure. For example, pathologists can diagnose Alzheimer's disease by observing plaques and tangles in the brain during an autopsy, but the ability to diagnose Alzheimer's disease this way isn't of particular value during someone's lifetime. In this case, researchers have a good gold standard, but for most studies they would need to use some way to diagnose the disease in a live patient.

Consequently, usually researchers must use some "less-than-gold standard," which may not perfectly represent the characteristic or disorder but at least provides some challenge to the validity of the diagnosis or measurement of interest. For instance, in Example 8.1, researchers used careful and multiple measurements of children's height made by trained and experienced pediatric endocrine nurses using precise equipment as a "less-than-gold" standard to compare the standard measurements made in the doctors' office.

Just as there are many types of reliability, there are many types of validity. Researchers will speak of face validity, construct validity, convergent validity, discriminative validity, predictive validity, and so on. The type of validity researchers consider depends on which less-than-gold standard they use as the criterion against which they evaluate the measure. The actual definitions of these different types of validity also vary from researcher to researcher. However, how a researcher names the type of validity is not as important as which gold standard (or "less-than-gold standard") they select for comparison. Usually, a correlation coefficient between the measurement or diagnosis in question and the gold standard is the coefficient of validity. That is, for a sample from the relevant population, researchers measure the characteristic using the method in question and using the method defined by the gold standard, each done "blinded" to the other. Then they calculate the correlation between the two different measures. Consider Example 8.6, which describes poor validity.

EXAMPLE 8.6

After surgery, patients typically self-assess their surgical wound for signs of infection. One study checked the validity of this method by following 290 patients for six weeks postoperatively. Infection control nurses also photographed their wounds and checked them for signs of infection. The correlation between the nurses' assessments and the patients were "low": 0.37. Interestingly, the correlation between the nurses' assessments and physicians' assessments of the photographs were only "moderate" (0.54).[7]

Consider also Example 8.7, which describes assessing validity with respect to obesity.

EXAMPLE 8.7

Estimating the reliability of the various methods to measure obesity as described in Example 8.4 is relatively easy. More difficult is estimating the validity of any one of these methods. For example, even though repeated skin-fold measurements produce similar results, how well do these skin-fold measurements measure an individual's true body composition? In particular, which other measure should be used as a "gold standard" to which to compare a particular measure? The accepted "gold standard" for obesity has changed over time from hydrostatic weighing[8] to various imaging technologies [e.g., magnetic resonance imaging (MRI), computer tomography (CT), and dual-energy X-ray absorptiometry (DEXA)].[9] For example, one researcher estimated the correlation between skin-fold measurements and hydrostatic weighing as 0.931 while the correlation between the impedance method and hydrostatic weighing was 0.830,[8] indicating that if hydrostatic weighing is an appropriate gold standard, these other two methods have high validity. Other researchers, however, who used direct measurement of fat tissue from dissected cadavers as a gold standard for comparison for skin-fold measurements have suggested that skin-fold measurements are not quite so valid.[10]

Often we have a tendency to believe that the more technologically advanced a measurement, the more valid or reliable it is. As shown in Example 8.7, measurements of obesity range from simple measures such as BMI and skin-folds to various imaging technologies, such as MRIs or DEXA. However, how technologically advanced a measure is does not necessarily correspond to how valid or reliable it is. With respect to obesity, for example, unpublished data suggest that the best predictor of mortality among women older than 65 is BMI, not some of the other more expensive, more difficult, and more technically advanced measures.[11,12] This result may not necessarily indicate that BMI is a more valid measure (since the outcome was death rather than some other measure of obesity), but it probably does indicate that BMI is a high-quality measure in this particular population.

Researchers typically demonstrate validity by showing that the measure closely matches a gold standard. However, one type of validity—face validity—is an exception to this rule. Face validity means simply that the measurement or diagnosis appears at "face value" to measure what it intends to measure or diagnose. For face validity, researchers need only provide a compelling argument that a measurement measures what it seems to measure. For example, few would disagree that checking a birth certificate for a person's date of birth and then subtracting that from today's date has face validity for determining someone's age. For many of the potential risk factors and outcomes in risk estimation, face validity is all that researchers demonstrate, and often all they need to demonstrate.

What Researchers Can Do to Improve Validity and Reliability

The reason we tend to hear more about the reliability of a measurement or a diagnosis than validity is because reliability is easier to measure and document, but perhaps more important, researchers often can directly improve reliability but usually can only improve validity by improving reliability. Recall that validity is part of reliability—validity measures the relevant information, and reliability measures the relevant and irrelevant information. As Figure 8.5 illustrates, efforts to improve reliability—that is, efforts that increase the amount of variability in a measurement or diagnosis that can be attributed to an individual or, equivalently, efforts that decrease random errors—often improve validity as well.

Often random error arises because of a lack of standardization in the measurement protocol. For example, in an IQ test, researchers can reduce random error by making sure the testing is done in a reasonably controlled environment. There should be no jackhammers outside the testing room window, nor should those taking the tests be required to sit at desks too small for them, nor should the exams be scheduled over mealtimes without recess. Similarly, many blood and urine tests are taken first thing in the morning after a night of fasting. Such protocol requirements improve the reliability of the measure. For example, in Example 8.1, researchers provided better equipment and trained primary care practice staff to take repeated measures and average them, remove a child's shoes, and so on, in an effort to improve the reliability of their measurements. In improving the reliability, they

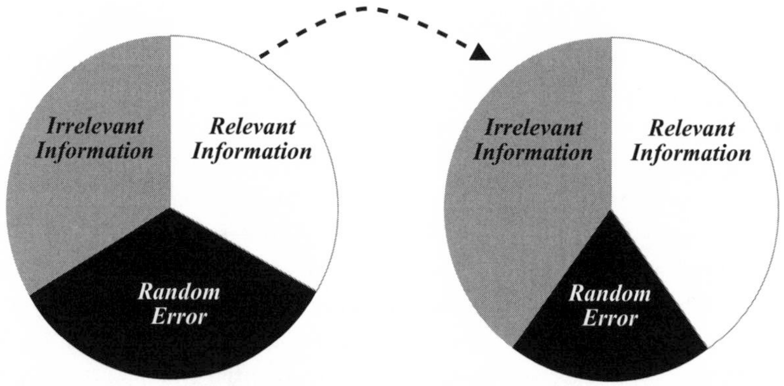

Figure 8.5. How decreasing random error typically improves both reliability and validity.

improved the validity of the measurements taken in the practitioners office as measured by how well the measurements matched the "expert" nurses.[2]

As the researchers demonstrated when they improved height measurement by having staff members measure and remeasure a child and average the results, usually taking three or more independent measurements and averaging them substantially increases the reliability.[13,14] For this reason, assays of body tissues (e.g., blood tests) are often done in triplicate and the average or median value used. Similarly, diagnoses can be improved by having more than one doctor make the diagnosis and then using some sort of strategy to "average" the diagnoses, such as having multiple diagnosticians confer and come to a consensus diagnosis. Consider Example 8.8.

EXAMPLE 8.8

An article titled "How Many Raters Are Needed for a Reliable Diagnosis?" describes how researchers studied how many consenting evaluators were necessary to achieve a reliability of 60% for various psychiatric disorders.[15] For example, to achieve a better than 60% reliability for diagnosing depression, they found that a consensus of three evaluators was necessary. Two evaluators were necessary for 60% reliability in diagnosing schizophrenia or neuroses, and more than three for personality disorder.

Consider another example of how researchers might improve reliability and validity. One of the most problematic situations is when risk factor measurement or outcome diagnosis is based on informants' reports. This strategy is most common when dealing with young children or with the seriously ill, who in many cases cannot report on themselves. In such cases, a common alternative is to query a mother or teacher about the child or a caregiver about the seriously ill, as well as obtaining a self-report where possible. Such reports are often quite reliable but have questionable validity since they frequently consist of information about both the informant (here irrelevant) and the individual (here relevant). Consequently, when researchers use multiple informants for the same individual, the informants often correlate poorly with each other.

To deal with this problem, researchers have realized that what an informant reports reflects not only the individual's trait of interest, but the context in which the informant observes the individual (e.g., home for the mother vs. school for the teacher), the perspective of the informant (i.e., reporting on self or on another), and of course, random error. If researchers mix and match informants, so that the perspectives and/or contexts overlap, then they are able to disentangle the trait of interest from the contexts and perspectives. For example, if researchers were interested about some characteristic of a school-age child, they might ask the child, the mother, and the teacher. In this case, there are two contexts (home, school) and two perspectives (self, other). Figure 8.6 depicts how two informants (the child and the mother) see the same context (home), while two informants (the mother and the teacher) have the same perspective (other). From this information, researchers can isolate the contribution from each perspective and each context, and then calculate appropriate weights to average the multiple informants' reports.[16]

Although we skip the statistical details of how the contexts and perspectives are disentangled (see reference 16), our point is that improving reliability and validity is a challenging problem, sometimes to be solved with innovative techniques.

On the other hand, sometimes researchers themselves reduce reliability and validity. The most common example occurs when researchers dichotomize an otherwise valid and reliable measurement. For example, for many years, cancer treatment was considered a success if the patient survived five years postdiagnosis and a failure otherwise. What that meant was that the treatment outcome of a patient who survived five years plus one day was considered the same as that of one who survived for 30 years postdiagnosis. But the outcome for a patient who died one day short of five years was considered completely different from that for a patient who died one day after five years. This doesn't make common sense, and makes for loss of reliability and validity, as well. When researchers suppress real variability among the individuals (here the variability in survival time) by grouping very different outcomes, the variability remains in the population, but the measurement

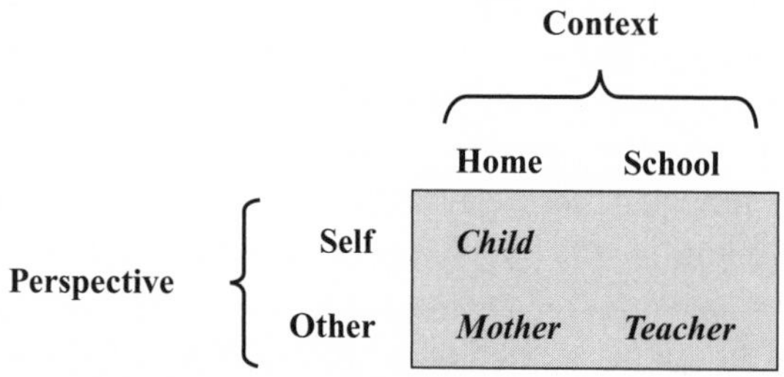

Figure 8.6. The overlap in perspective and context when three different informants are used: the child, the mother, and the teacher. The child's perspective is himself or herself, and the context is home. The mother's perspective is nonself (other), but her perspective is also home. Finally, the teacher's perspective is also other, but his or her perspective is school.

ignores it. The net result is that the circle in Figure 8.1 is partitioned differently—the suppressed variability is routed into the error, decreasing reliability and validity. Fortunately, in recent years cancer trials have tended to report survival curves, thus using the entire time continuum rather than using an arbitrary dichotomization of time.

This warning against dichotomization might seem contrary to our previous discussion about outcomes and potency. We say outcomes for risk estimation are binary, and we say that in order to calculate potency we determine a high-risk group and a low-risk group and compare how many in each group have the outcome. Determining a high-risk and a low-risk group requires dichotomization of a risk factor—that is, selecting a cutoff typically above which people are considered high risk and below which people are considered low risk. Moreover, we argued such a dichotomization was necessary to facilitate both policy and clinical decision making. However, we advocate such dichotomization *once the research is concluded and the issue moves toward medical decision making.* Once a measurement of either a risk factor or the outcome is dichotomized, some of the information contained in that measure is essentially thrown away. Such an action should not be taken until after the analysis phase of a research project. That is, for example, researchers should not merely record whether or not a cancer patient survived more than five years; they should record how long the cancer patient survived. Later, if necessary for communication or other purposes, an optimal cutoff can be determined by comparing the potency of many cutoffs.

Conclusion and Summary

What is important about validity and reliability of measurement, particularly to medical decision makers? When considering a research result for risk estimation, we have already stressed the importance of checking the population studied, checking for statistically significant results and potency, and carefully scrutinizing how a study is designed. Reliability and validity of the measurements, however, are often not at the forefront of criticism of a result, nor do researchers typically report the reliability and validity of the measures they used.

When two different studies report different findings even with a similar research design and a similar population, the difference could be due to differences in the reliability and validity of the measurements or diagnoses. When researchers report nonstatistically significant results, the explanation could be poor reliability of the risk factor measurement or of the diagnosis.

Anyone evaluating the result of a risk estimation study needs to carefully examine how the diagnosis is made and how the risk factors are measured, by whom, and under what circumstances. Although typically not a lot of information about validity and reliability is provided in journal articles, researchers should provide some assurance that they measured the risk factors and outcome both reliably and validly. Often we assume that the more technically advanced the measurement or diagnosis is, the "better" it is. For example, lately we hear about a lot of imaging technologies, brain scans, and so on. Until researchers conduct and publish studies describing the validity and reliability of these measures, however, we don't know whether they are truly better than the less technical measurements already in use.

- The variability in a measurement or diagnosis can be attributed to relevant information, irrelevant information, and random error.
- The validity of a measurement or a diagnosis is the proportion of a measurement's/diagnosis's variability that is attributable to relevant information in a specified population. That is, how well does in a specified population does the measure or diagnosis represent the characteristic or disorder of interest?
- The reliability of a measurement or a diagnosis is the proportion of the variability of a measurement or diagnosis that is not due to random error or, alternatively, how well researchers can reproduce a measurement/diagnosis on repeated trials in a specified population.
- Poor reliability and validity may result in the inability to demonstrate that a real effect exists. Results that are not statistically significant may be due to poor reliability or validity of the measures used rather than the possibility that the hypothesis was wrong. Poor reliability and validity may also attenuate potency.
- Typically, researchers assess reliability by calculating a correlation coefficient between more than one independent measure or diagnosis (a "reliability coefficient").
- Typically, researchers assess validity by calculating a correlation coefficient between the measure of interest and another measure considered a "gold standard."
- Improving reliability and validity is primarily achieved by reducing sources of random error. Such practices include careful standardization of testing or diagnostic procedures, training of assessors, or using consensus measurements or diagnoses.
- Anyone intending to use the results of a risk estimation needs to consider whether the measures of either the potential risk factor or of the outcome were reliably and validly measured.

III

Cutting-Edge Approaches

The topics in Parts I and II—clear and precise terminology, how to recognize which risk factors are important, how risk factors work together to produce an outcome, and how to recognize good and bad research—were directed toward a broad audience with the goal of motivating all of us to use more precise language and demand better research and better communication of that research.

Part III presents methodology to help accomplish the goal of producing better research. Because Part III focuses specifically on research methodology, we direct it primarily toward researchers. Two of the topics—how strong the risk factor is (Chapter 9) and how we do moderator–mediator analysis (Chapter 10)—we have already discussed in nontechnical terms in Chapters 4 and 5. In Chapter 9, first we compare and contrast the different available measures of potency to support our recommendation that measuring the clinical significance of a risk factor requires consideration of the benefit of correctly predicting an outcome versus the harm of incorrectly predicting an outcome. We then illustrate how to select the most potent risk factor from a list of many. However, researchers' goals are not simply to select the most potent risk factor, particularly since often individual risk factors *by themselves* are not very potent. Thus, in Chapter 10, we will consider multiple risk factors.

Specifically, methodologically, how do researchers pare down and sort a long list of risk factors by identifying moderators and mediators, as well as proxy, independent, and overlapping risk factors?

Finally, after addressing how we should think about multiple risk factors, we return to the topic of potency with respect to multiple risk factors (Chapter 11). Specifically, how should we use multiple risk factors? Having a better understanding of how multiple risk factors work together is instructive from a theoretical standpoint, but when practitioners need to know exactly who has highest and who has lowest risk, understanding the interrelationships between the risk factors does not always help. Instead, practitioners need to know how to actually estimate risk for different groups of people depending on their profile of risk factors. To this task, we present a methodology to determine the highest and lowest risk groups using multiple risk factors.

Our goal for Part III is to provide the researcher with the methodological tools to help accomplish some of the challenges we argue researchers must overcome in order to produce results more relevant to medical decision making.

Although we believe much of the information presented in these chapters should be accessible and may be quite interesting to those not directly involved in conducting risk research, some may wish to skip to Chapter 12, where we summarize briefly the contents of these and all previous chapters. The last two chapters of this book (Chapters 13 and 14) are again directed to all readers and do not assume the reader has read all of Part III.

9

How Strong Is the Risk Factor?

Potency

An old saying asserts that the common cold usually lasts about seven days if you treat it, and about a week if you don't. This saying acknowledges that even with the "treatments" available, whether pharmaceutical, herbal, or chicken soup, nothing really changes the course of the illness. Luckily, most of these available remedies don't cause harm and may at least bring some level of comfort. Colds are usually short-lived and aren't really worth subjecting yourself to any treatment that might be worse than having the cold in the first place. The same is hardly true of other disorders—particularly ones such as cancer or heart disease that lead to disability or death, or psychiatric disorders that compromise normal functioning and quality of life. For such disorders, we are less willing to do nothing. But how do we know when an intervention (prevention or treatment) might be worse than the disorder itself? How can a researcher determine and communicate how much a risk factor matters when used either to identify who should receive an intervention or as the basis of an intervention?

In Chapter 4, we stressed that some relationship, no matter how small, probably exists between most factors and most subsequent outcomes. For researchers to establish a risk factor, they must first demonstrate that a "statistically significant" relationship exists between a preceding factor and an outcome. After all, if they can't even show convincing evidence that the risk factor is any better than flipping a coin or using a random number to make decisions, how useful can it be? But the researchers' job does not end there. In addition, they should evaluate and communicate the risk factor's clinical significance. Researchers measure clinical significance by measuring potency—a measure of how much better than random, and how much worse than perfect, a risk factor identifies who will have a particular outcome.

In this chapter, we expand the discussion of potency in Chapter 4 by comparing and contrasting some of the most common measures as well as justifying our own recommendation for the weighted kappa coefficient.

We Must Consider Both the Harm and Benefits of Using Risk Factors

The benefits of risk researchers' findings are easy to acknowledge: identifying risk factors, using these risk factors both to identify people who are at high risk for the outcome, and possibly intervening upon such risk factors to improve the outcome. But there is another side of the coin that is often overlooked: among those who are identified as high risk, some may never develop the outcome (false positives). Similarly, some identified as low risk will develop the outcome (false negatives). Intervening on those identified as high risk may not prevent the disorder—the benefit may be limited. Intervening unnecessarily on those incorrectly identified as high risk may do harm.

Imagine if you were told that you were at high risk of developing Alzheimer's disease in the next 10 years. Currently, there is nothing that can be done to prevent or delay this disease—thus, no benefit results from this information. But think of the harm if this information were wrong! The quality of your life may suffer from the anxiety and worry of what is predicted, completely unnecessarily.

Likewise, consider the currently available genetic test for Huntington's disease. This crippling disease strikes people in their 30s and 40s and eventually (painfully and slowly) leads to dementia and death. Like Alzheimer's, currently there is no cure and no way to delay its onset. Some people with a family history of the disease choose not to take the test—for them the harm of knowing outweighs the benefit. Others see more benefit in taking the test: if they test negative they ameliorate their worries about the future; if they test positive, they can prepare their families financially and psychologically. Again, suppose the test were wrong. Some people might choose not to have children in order to avoid passing on the disease. They might be reluctant to make any long-range plans, living from year to year, knowing that their life will be cut short.

Finally, recall our discussion on prostate-specific antigen (PSA) tests for prostate cancer. The benefit of true positives is to identify men who should undergo biopsies to detect prostate cancer early before the cancer spreads and becomes fatal. The harm of false positives, however, is that some men will undergo biopsies that detect no cancers at all. In addition, some of the biopsies might discover prostate cancers that would have never spread or otherwise impact normal functioning. These men, however, may still get treatment and possibly end up incontinent and impotent.

Determining statistical significance is easy. For example, repeated studies have demonstrated the statistically significant relationship between PSA level and prostate cancer. On the other hand, determining the clinical significance of risk factors is very complex, depending on far more than simply being able to determine who is at high risk and who is at low risk. When a risk factor is used to split a population into a high-risk group and a low-risk group, there are four resulting possibilities: true positives and true negatives, false positives and false negatives. These four possibilities are illustrated in Figure 9.1, as well as indications of when benefits and harms might result. What those benefits and harms are vary from one situation to another, because every outcome in every population has its own unique set of concerns.

Notice that the probabilities of true negatives, false positives, false negatives, and true positives all depend on the values of sensitivity (Se) and specificity (Sp). Researchers often use sensitivity and specificity as potency measures themselves, but they also use them to calculate the values of other potency measures.

> *Sensitivity (Se): In a particular population, the probability that someone who will have the outcome is classified as* high *risk.*

> *Specificity (Sp): In a particular population, the probability that someone who will* not *have the outcome is classified as* low *risk.*

Put another way, sensitivity measures the probability of true positives among those who will have the outcome, while specificity measures the probability of true negatives among those who will not have the outcome. When we're looking at harm versus benefits of using risk factors, we are usually considering true positives (benefit) and false positives (harm). While sensitivity is related to benefits (i.e., true positives), one minus specificity—the probability of false positives among those who will not have the outcome—is related to harm. We discuss sensitivity and specificity (or one minus

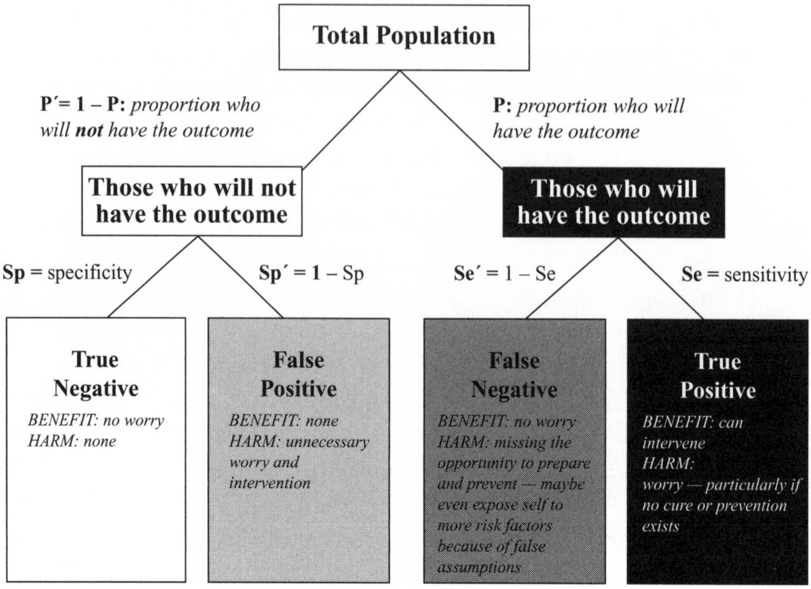

Figure 9.1. The four possible outcomes when a risk factor is used to split a population into a high-risk and a low-risk group.

specificity) extensively in this chapter, particularly when we introduce the receiver operating characteristic (ROC) approach.

An easy way to remember sensitivity and specificity (and which is which) is to consider an airport metal detector. When the detector is very sensitive, it sounds an alarm for someone's belt buckle, bracelet, pocket change, and so on. Being so *sensitive,* the metal detectors are very likely to "catch" someone carrying a metal weapon (true positives). However, in doing so, there are going to be many false alarms (false positives). Many false positives means that the metal detector has *low* specificity—the metal detector is not being very specific to the weapons it is trying to detect. Typically sensitivity and specificity "see-saw"—the more sensitive a risk factor, the less specific, and conversely, the more specific a risk factor, the less sensitive.

Using sensitivity and specificity, researchers can easily calculate the proportion of the population who may potentially experience harm or benefit, but quantifying how much "good" to attribute to that benefit and how much "bad" to attribute to that harm is not as simple. How should researchers present potency in a way that is amenable to determining the clinical significance? Many potency measures exist, but they do not all communicate clinical significance in the same ways. In Table 9.1, for example, we list several measures of potency that we discussed in this book. Many of these measures have additional variants—for example, three other measures of potency (log odds ratio, Yule's index, and gamma) are simply rescalings of the odds ratio (OR), one of the most commonly used potency measures.

As we said before, the problem with having so many different potency measures is knowing which one best communicates the clinical significance of a risk factor. Also, if all these measures are computed differently and are calibrated to have different values for random and perfect association, which one should we be familiar with to comprehend a risk factor's potency? Finally, how do we respond when some measures of potency suggest a risk factor is potent, while others do not? Consider Example 9.1.

EXAMPLE 9.1

Suppose researchers have an intervention targeted at preventing schizophrenia. In addition, they have a risk factor to identify those at high risk for schizophrenia who might benefit from an intervention. For this example, let's assume that those identified by the risk factor as high risk who will actually develop schizophrenia (the true positives) will benefit from the intervention, while those identified as high risk who will not develop schizophrenia (the false positives) will be harmed by being subjected to the intervention unnecessarily. Figure 9.2 depicts a 2 × 2 table of association between a risk factor and an outcome, defining some of the probabilities (Q, P, Se, and Sp) that we will use to calculate one of the most commonly used measures of potency, the odds ratio.

The proportion of the population who will benefit from having a risk factor to identify those who are high risk for schizophrenia is the prevalence of schizophrenia times the sensitivity ($P \cdot \text{Se}$), and the proportion who will be harmed is the proportion of the population who will *not* develop schizophrenia ($1 - P = P'$) times one minus the specificity ($P' \cdot \text{Sp}'$). [Note: P can denote either the prevalence or the incidence, depending on whether the outcome is defined as a prevalence or an incidence outcome. For convenience in this discussion, we will call P the prevalence.]

Suppose the prevalence (P) of schizophrenia in a population is 1%, and the sensitivity and the specificity of this risk factor for schizophrenia are both 80% (i.e., $\text{Sp} = \text{Se} = 0.8$). With this information and some algebra, we can calculate the odds ratio [$\text{OR} = AD/BC = (\text{Se} \cdot \text{Sp})/(\text{Se}' \cdot \text{Sp}') = 16$]. Typically, researchers interpret a risk factor with an odds ratio

Table 9.1
Some Existing Measures of Potency

Measure	Mathematical Definition	Random Value	Perfect Value
Measures used as potency measures themselves, but also used in mathematical definitions below			
Sensitivity	A/P	Q	1
Specificity	D/P'	Q'	1
Positive predictive value	$PVP = A/Q$	P	1
Negative predictive value	$PVN = D/Q'$	P'	1
Measures commonly used and to be discussed			
Risk difference (I and II)[a]	I: $Se + Sp - 1$ II: $PVP + PVN - 1$	0	1
Odds ratio[b]	$(AD)/(BC)$ or $(Se \cdot Sp)/(Se' \cdot Sp)$	1	∞
Risk ratio (I and II)[b]	I: $Se/(1 - Sp)$ II: $Sp/(1 - Se)$	1	∞
Risk ratio (III and IV)[b]	III: $PVP/(1 - PVN)$ IV: $PVN/(1 - PVP)$	1	∞
Phi coefficient	$\varphi = PP'(Se - Sp')/(PP'QQ')^{1/2}$	0	1
Weighted kappa	$\kappa(r) = PP'(Se - Sp')/(PQ'r + P'Qr')$	0	1
Number needed to take	$1/(PVP + PVN - 1)$	∞	1

[a]Also referred to as Youden's index.
[b]Both the odds ratio and the four different risk ratios are sometimes also referred to as "relative risk."

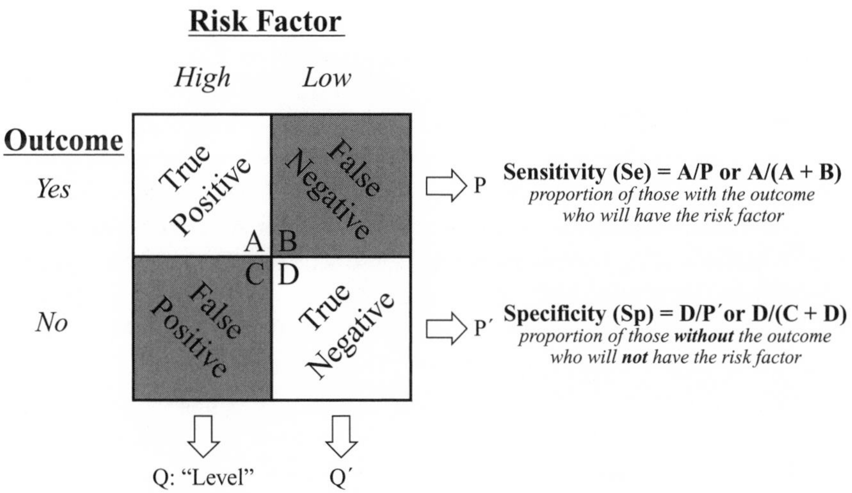

Figure 9.2. A 2 × 2 table of association between a risk factor and an outcome. *A* is the probability of a true positive, *B* of a false negative, *C* of a false positive, and *D* of a true negative. *P* is the prevalence of the outcome, and *Q* is the "level" of the risk factor—that is, the proportion of the population that will be considered high risk.

of 16 as a very potent risk factor, and they would probably report it as a "highly statistically significant" risk factor. However, in this case, of every 1,000 people, $1{,}000 \cdot P' \cdot Sp' = 1{,}000 \cdot 0.99 \cdot 0.20 = 198$ people would be harmed to every $1{,}000 \cdot P \cdot Se = 1{,}000 \cdot 0.01 \cdot 0.80 = 8$ people benefited. Alternatively said, the harm-to-benefit ratio is 198/8 = 24.75, or about 25 people are harmed to every one person who benefits.

In contrast, suppose that 50% of a population is likely to develop schizophrenia ($P = 0.50$), and the sensitivity and specificity are still each 80%. The odds ratio is still 16, and the risk factor is still likely to be reported as highly statistically significant. But now for every 1,000 people, $1{,}000 \cdot 0.2 \cdot 0.5 = 100$ people are harmed and $1{,}000 \cdot 0.5 \cdot 0.8 = 400$ people are benefited—that is, the harm-to-benefit ratio is 0.25. The odds ratio has not changed; the clinical significance certainly has.

The message of Example 9.1 is that to examine the clinical significance of a risk factor, we must consider and acknowledge both the possible benefit and the harm. Simply knowing the commonly reported odds ratio is not enough. The cases described in Example 9.1 both have an odds ratio of 16.0, but in one case 25 people were harmed for every one benefited, and in the other case, four people benefited for every one harmed. If the intervention is one where the harm was negligible and benefit considerable, perhaps a harm-to-benefit ratio of 25 is fine and 0.25 even better, but if the intervention is one where the harm is considerable and the benefit moderate, that would be a very different story.

As Table 9.1 shows, however, the odds ratio is only one of many available measures. In the next section, we introduce a visual way to compare and contrast some of the more common measures of potency. With this visual method, the ROC approach,[1] we plot the sensitivity (Se) of a risk factor against one minus its specificity (1 – Sp or, equivalently, Sp'). With a little experience and understanding of a few specific characteristics of the plot, we can easily look at points corresponding to different risk factors and see how they differ in potency. In addition, by using such a plot, we can illustrate what each of the existing measures of potency actually measures and see if and when these measures fail to convey important information.

What Is the Receiver Operator Characteristic Approach?

When we give someone directions to some unfamiliar location, we often draw a map. We highlight particular landmarks to help someone see where that unfamiliar location is relative to more familiar or recognizable sites on the map. Plotting the sensitivity and one minus the specificity of a risk factor in an ROC plot (or equivalently described as the "ROC plane") is similar to drawing a map and marking the places of interest. For linguistic simplicity, we'll describe this plotting of the sensitivity and one minus the specificity of a risk factor as "locating the risk factor" and the point corresponding to a risk factor as the "location of the risk factor."

Before we can begin "reading" this map, let's highlight the "landmarks"—the particular fixed features that are easy to identify and help you to get your bearings. Then we can discuss different points on this map corresponding to different risk factors relative to these landmarks. The ROC plane (see Figure 9.3) has two such landmarks, a line called the random ROC and a point called the ideal point.

The *random ROC* is the diagonal line from the bottom left corner of the plot to the upper right corner. Points located on this line correspond to random decision making—that is, deciding who is at high risk and who is at low risk by flipping a coin, tossing a die, or simply making a completely uneducated guess. Specifically, this line represents all points where the sensitivity is equal to one minus the specificity. In the appendix, we include a mathematical demonstration of why the sensitivity equals one minus the specificity for random decision making. In that demonstration, we also show that the percent-

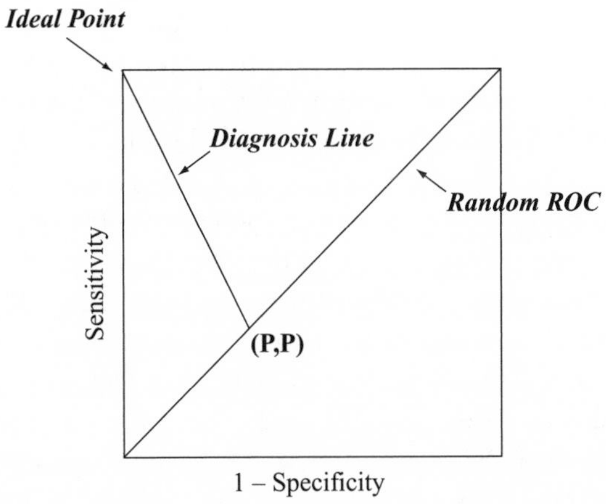

Figure 9.3. The ROC plane. Risk factors located on the random ROC line correspond to random decision making. A risk factor that perfectly predicts the outcome would be located at the ideal point. The diagnosis line connects the ideal point to the random ROC at the point (P, P). Measures of potency measure the distance a risk factor lies from the random ROC line and/or from the ideal point. The diagnosis line serves as a "compass" to allow you to see how the level of the risk factor (Q) compares to the prevalence of the outcome (P).

age of people labeled "high risk" by the random decision (referred to as the level or Q) is also equal to the sensitivity and to one minus the specificity.

A true risk factor cannot actually be located on the random ROC since by our definition a risk factor must be nonrandomly associated with the outcome. However, risk factors can lie very close to the random ROC, indicating they are not much better than random decision making. Suppose your doctor walks into the examining room, and, instead of reading your medical chart or examining you, she or he pulls out a quarter and flips it. Heads, you'll receive medication (or surgery—take your choice of painful and possibly harmful interventions!); tails, you won't. That would be ridiculous—but equivalent to using a factor that is only randomly associated with the outcome. Instead, suppose your doctor orders a battery of medical tests costing many thousands of dollars, but suppose those tests located in the ROC plane are not far from the random ROC. Then the decision to prescribe medication or perform surgery based on those tests might be even more ridiculous, little better than tossing that quarter. Thus, to evaluate potency is to look at how much better a risk factor is than flipping a coin and deciding whether it's worth the costs and consequences the subsequent decisions might have.

The first thing we look at when evaluating the potency of risk factors using this methodology is how far it is from the random ROC. However, we will also be concerned about measuring the distance of the risk factor to the other "landmark" in the ROC plane, the *ideal point.* The ideal point is the point in the upper left hand corner where sensitivity equals one (i.e., no false negatives) and the specificity is one (i.e., no false positives). In other words, a risk factor, if one existed, located at the ideal point perfectly predicts the outcome. Different measures of potency are actually different ways of measuring a risk factor's distance to the random ROC and/or to the ideal point.

In addition to landmarks, a map includes a compass—some symbol indicating which direction is north, south, east, and west. The corresponding reference in the ROC "map" is referred to as the *diagnosis line* (the name is a relic from the ROC's original application in medicine for medical test evaluation). The diagnosis line connects the ideal point and the point (P, P), where P is the proportion of the population who will have the outcome. When the level of the risk factor (Q = proportion of people classified as high risk) is the same as P, the risk factor must lie on that diagnosis line. Any risk factor that characterizes a proportion Q as high risk other than P lies on a line parallel to the diagnosis line, cutting the random ROC at the point (Q, Q). (A mathematical demonstration of this is included in the appendix.) Thus, when we locate a risk factor in the ROC plane, the distance from this point to the diagnosis line reflects the difference between Q and P. We can "read off" the level Q by drawing a line parallel to the diagnosis line from the risk factor to the random ROC. The point (Q, Q) is where the line hits the random ROC.

Just as a compass is critical for understanding which direction you are going, the diagnosis line is critical for visually comprehending the prevalence P of the outcome and how that prevalence compares to the level Q of each risk factor under consideration. As Example 9.1 illustrated, P and Q along with sensitivity and specificity are requisite for calculating the proportion benefited and harmed by using a risk factor to predict an outcome. Thus, although different measures of potency are different ways of measuring a risk factor's distance to the "landmarks" (the random ROC and the ideal point), how this distance is measured must somehow incorporate the diagnosis line (i.e., P and Q) to also capture the benefits and harms of true positives and false positives.

To compare several measures of potency, in Example 9.2 we use data from the Infant Health and Development Program (IHDP). The IHDP was an eight-site randomized clinical trial evaluating the efficacy of an early intervention program to improve the health and functioning of low-birth-weight premature children.[2] We will locate risk factors identified in this study to learn more about the ROC approach, to illustrate locating risk factors in the ROC plane, and finally to illustrate selecting the most potent risk factor. [Note: This is strictly demonstration. If we were really analyzing these data, we would include many more potential risk factors, e.g., gender and site.]

EXAMPLE 9.2

In Figure 9.4 we plot sensitivities and one minus the specificities of three risk factors for low IQ identified in the control group of the IHDP study. Children in this control group received good-quality standard medical follow-up but no novel intervention. Researchers used a low IQ at age three defined by a Stanford-Binet score lower than 85 as an early indicator of poor school readiness.

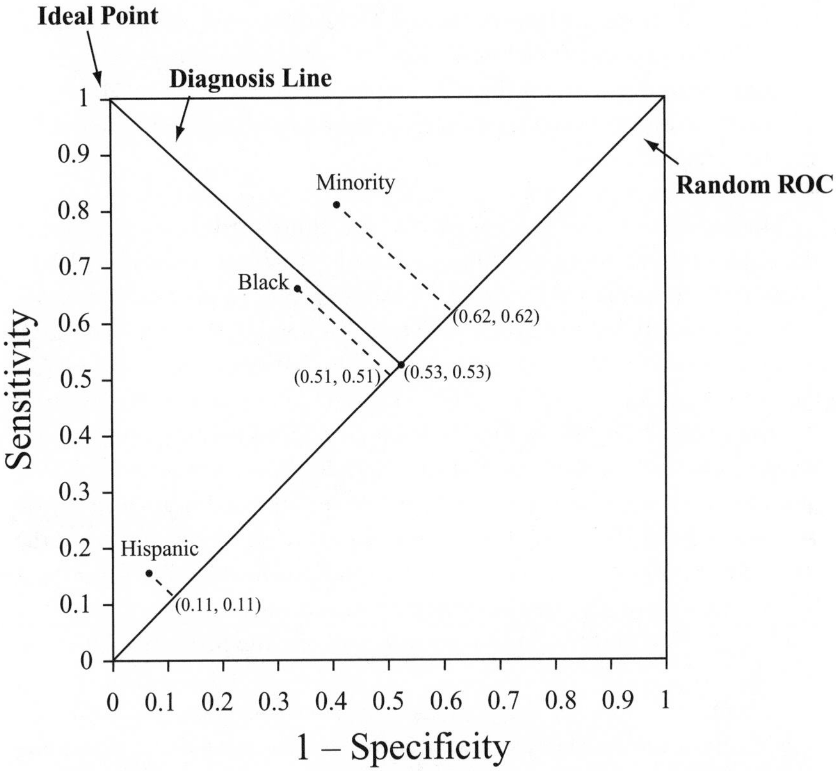

Figure 9.4. The locations in the ROC plane of three risk factors for low IQ from the IHDP data. The dotted lines indicate how the level (Q) of each risk factor (i.e., the proportion of self-reported Hispanics, blacks, and minorities) can be "read off" the plot by drawing a line parallel to the diagnosis line and seeing where it hits the random ROC line.

The three plotted risk factors are self-reports of being black (Sp' = 0.34, Se = 0.67), Hispanic (Sp' = 0.06, Se = 0.16), or either black or Hispanic (Sp' = 0.40, Se = 0.82)—we label the last risk factor as "minority."

The first thing we locate on this plot is the diagnosis line. A large percentage (53%) of the children in this population of low-birth-weight premature children have low IQ. Thus, $P = 0.53$, and the diagnosis line connects the ideal point with the point (P, P) or (0.53, 0.53). With the diagnosis line in place, we can easily "eyeball" the proportion of blacks, Hispanics, and minorities in the sample by drawing lines parallel to the diagnosis line from each of these points and seeing where they cross the random ROC. From this we can see that the levels (Q) of these risk factors are 0.51 (i.e., 51% of the sample are black), 0.11 (i.e., 11% of this sample are Hispanic), and 0.62 (i.e., 62% of the sample are minorities). Since the level of the risk factor "minority" is higher (62%) than the prevalence of low IQ ($P = 53\%$), it lies above the diagnosis line. Since the levels of the risk factors "black" (51%) and "Hispanic" (11%) are lower than the prevalence, these risk factors are located below the diagnosis line.

In Example 9.2, notice that each of the plotted risk factors lies above the random ROC. All risk factors associated with an increase in the likelihood of the outcome will lie above the random ROC. When having the risk factor is associated with a decrease in the likelihood of the outcome (i.e., a protective factor), the point corresponding to that risk factor will lie *below* the random ROC. However, we can always redefine such a risk factor as the absence of a protective factor. Then all points corresponding to risk factors for an outcome lie above the random ROC. For example, instead of plotting "exercising regularly" as a protective factor for heart disease, we can plot "*not* exercising regularly" as a risk factor. Then, the location of the risk factor moves from below the random ROC to above it. For simplification purposes, we will assume that all risk factors are located above the random ROC, or if they do not, we will redefine the protective factor so that they do.

Finally, after locating the three risk factors and the diagnosis line in the ROC plane as described in Example 9.2, we turn our attention to evaluating the potency of these three risk factors based on race/ethnicity. To do this, we will examine some of the most common ways researchers currently measure and report potency and demonstrate what distances, in the ROC plane, they are actually measuring.

The Risk Difference Does Not Consider the Prevalence of the Outcome

If we look at the three points on Figure 9.5 corresponding to black, Hispanic, and minority, we can see that Hispanic is closest to the random ROC and minority is farthest. This visual inspection produces the first measure of potency we will discuss, the *risk difference I* (Se – Sp'). [Note: The risk difference II is the same as risk difference I if we replace Se by positive predicted value (PVP) and Sp by negative predicted value (PVN).] The risk difference is simply proportional to the shortest distance between the plotted risk factor to the random ROC. For any point on the random ROC, the risk difference is zero, while for a point at the ideal point the risk difference is one. Thus, the risk difference ranges from zero (random) to one (perfect).

In the IHDP example (Example 9.2), the risk difference for Hispanic is 0.10, for black is 0.33, and for minority is 0.42. Thus, the minority risk

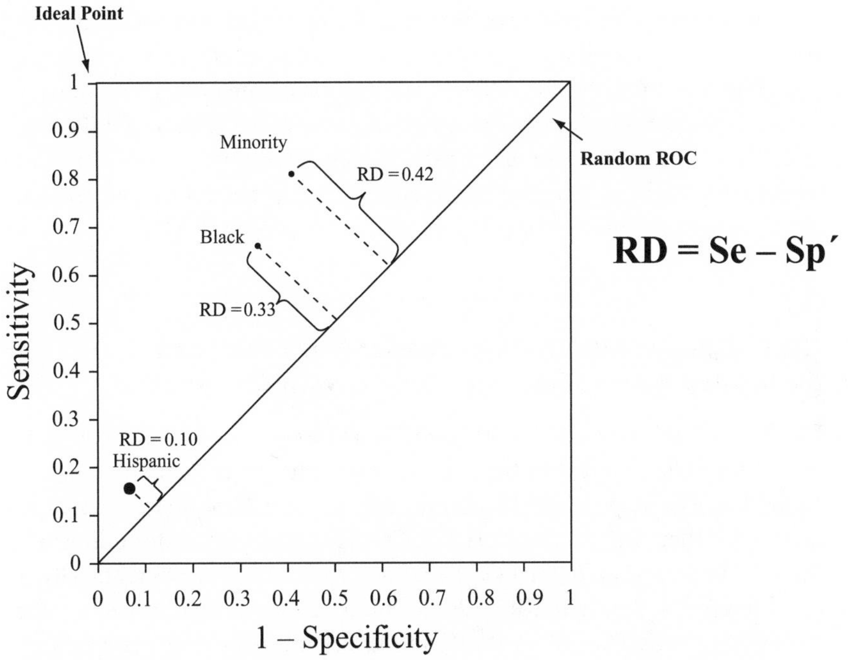

Figure 9.5. How the risk differences for three risk factors are measured in the ROC plane. Risk difference (RD) is the distance from the risk factor to the random ROC. Using the risk difference, minority is the most potent risk factor for low IQ in this population, and Hispanic is the least.

factor by this measure is considered the most potent. However, the risk difference is based only on distance from the random ROC and ignores how the prevalence (*P*) of the outcome compares to the level (*Q*) of the risk factor. Recall that the level of the risk factor Hispanic is 11% and the level of the risk factor minority is 62%. Remember that those levels will have bearing upon the harm benefit balance—the more people identified as high risk, the more potential for misidentifying, and possibly causing harm by treating unnecessarily.

In fact, any risk factor with *Q* either very near zero (e.g., Hispanic) or very near one must lie in one of the corners of the ROC plane at either end of the random ROC. In these corners, it is not possible to move too far away from the random ROC. Thus, risk factors that are rare (*Q* near zero) or very common (*Q* near one) are always going to have a risk difference near zero. But are these risk factors necessarily less important than others closer to the middle? For a rare disorder, does it make sense that a "good" risk factor identifies many people of high risk? Would you really want to treat 50% of the population for an outcome that only affects 1%?

Sometimes, but not always, the tendency of the risk difference to favor risk factors with a level (*Q*) near 50% is exactly what researchers want to do. Then and only then, the risk difference is an appropriate measure of potency to use. However, researchers can miscommunicate the clinical significance of a risk factor if they present a risk difference without consideration of whether this particular measure of potency is appropriate for the risk factors, outcome, and population of interest.

The Risk Ratios Also Do Not Consider Prevalence, and the Related Ratios Sometimes Conflict with One Another

Let us try a different tack: the *risk ratios.* Suppose we draw the lines connecting the point determined by the risk factor and the two corners, as shown in Figure 9.6. The slope of the line on the left is one risk ratio (RR_1) equal to Se/(1 – Sp) (here RR_1 = 1.9 for black, 2.6 for Hispanic, and 2.0 for minority); the slope of the line on the right is the *reciprocal* of the another risk ratio (RR_2) equal to Sp/(1 – Se) (here RR_2 = 2.0 for black, 1.1 for Hispanic, and 3.4 for minority). [Note: The risk ratios III and IV are the same as the risk ratios I and II if we replace Se by PVP and Sp by PVN.]

Any point related to a factor that lies directly on the random ROC has both slopes equal to one. Thus, both risk ratios for a risk factor near the random ROC are close to one. At the other extreme, any risk factor near the ideal point has both risk ratios near infinity. Thus, in contrast to the

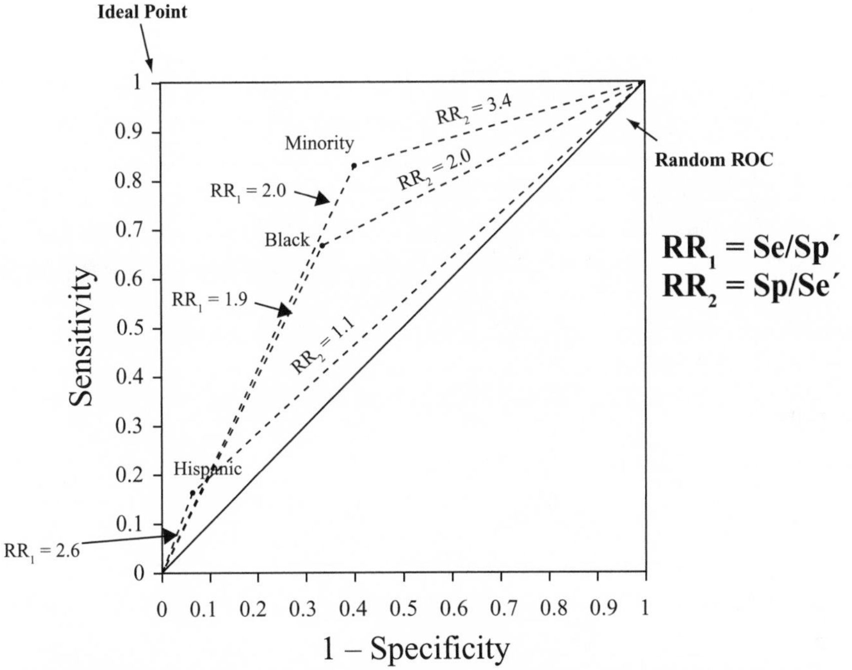

Figure 9.6. How risk ratios I and II for three risk factors are measured in the ROC plane. The slope of the line connecting the risk factor to the lower left corner is risk ratio I (RR_1). The slope of the line connecting the risk factor to the upper right corner is risk ratio II (RR_2). Using RR_1, Hispanic is the most potent risk factor, while using RR_2, minority is the most potent risk factor.

risk difference that ranges from zero to one, both risk ratios range from one to infinity.

Again, consider those two corners. In these corners, one of the risk ratios (the one corresponding to the longer line) may be near 1.0, suggesting random association, while the other (corresponding to the shorter line) may be very large, suggesting strong association. Which indication to believe is part of the problem of measuring potency using risk ratios. In the present case, Hispanic is the most potent risk factor when you consider RR_1, while minority is the most potent when you consider RR_2. How should researchers decide which risk ratio to use and which risk factor is more potent? If researchers are reporting the potency of a single risk factor, should they report RR_1 or RR_2?

Unfortunately, given that there are at least two different risk ratios and that they can give very different answers (as they often do), the risk ratio is a questionable choice as a measure of potency.

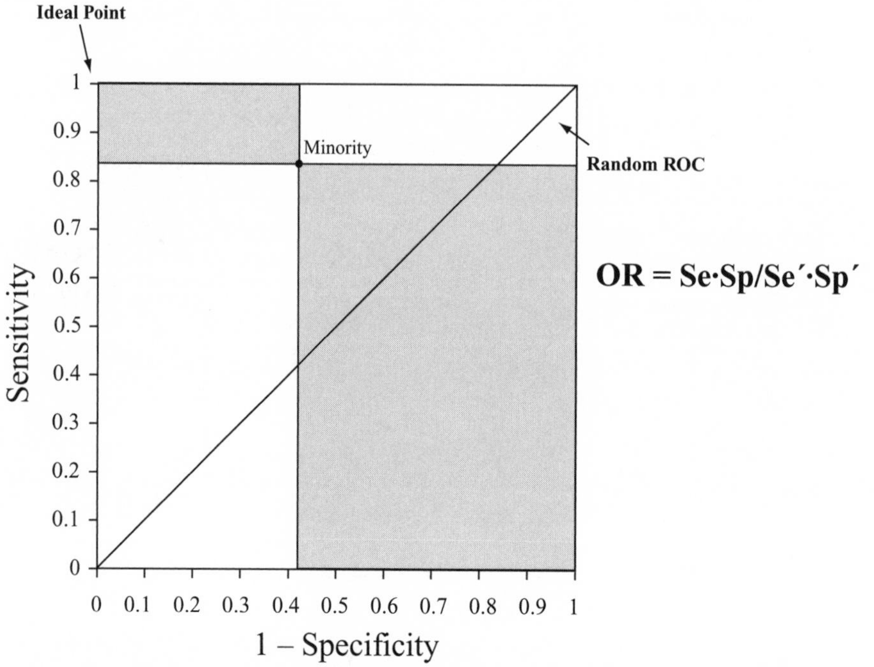

Figure 9.7. How the odds ratio for the risk factor minority is measured in the ROC plane. The odds ratio is the ratio of the area of the lower right box to the area of the upper left box, where each box is created by drawing "crosshairs" centered at the risk factor extending to the edges of the ROC plane.

The Odds Ratio Also Does Not Consider Prevalence

Let's try yet another tack: the *odds ratio.* While the risk difference and the risk ratios are both often seen in the risk research literature, the most commonly used measure of potency is the odds ratio. The odds ratio is a ratio of the areas of two "boxes" (Figure 9.7). The boxes are determined by drawing a vertical and a horizontal line through the location of the risk factor to the edges of the ROC plane. The ratio of the area of the lower right box to the upper left box is the odds ratio [OR = AD/BC or (Se·Sp)/(Se'·Sp')]. The odds ratio for black is 3.8, for Hispanic 2.8, and for minority 7.0.

For any point on the random ROC, the areas of the two boxes are the same, so the odds ratio is one. For any point near the ideal point, the upper box becomes very small with the area near zero, while the lower box is quite large, producing an odds ratio approaching infinity. Thus, like the two risk ratios, the odds ratio ranges from one to infinity. Moreover, the odds ratio actually equals the product of the two risk ratios, making it always bigger than the biggest risk ratio.

One of the major attractions of the odds ratio appears to be how big it is, even when the risk factor is only modestly above the random ROC. In Figure 9.8, we show curves ("equipotency curves") along each of which the value of the odds ratio is the same. Of course, along the random ROC, the odds ratio equals 1.0. Notice that even when the odds ratio is 2.2, it is barely above the random ROC. Yet the risk research literature is filled with statistically significant risk factors with odds ratios below 2.2. Note that *at best*—that is, at the peak of the curve—a point with odds ratio = 2.2 is 20% of the way between the random ROC and the ideal point. A point with odds ratio = 5.4 is *at best* 40% of the way; a point with odds ratio = 16.0 is *at best* 60% of

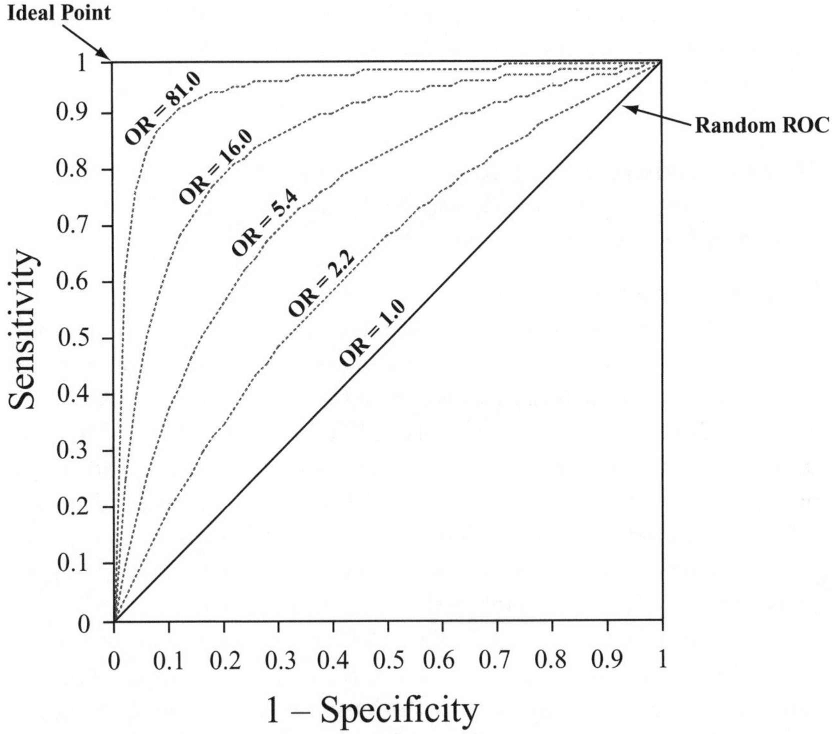

Figure 9.8. Equipotency curves for the odds ratio. The peaks of the five curves are 0%, 20%, 40%, 60%, and 80% along the way from the random ROC to the ideal point. Along each of these curves, the odds ratio is the same. Notice that an odds ratio of 2.2—usually considered a "large" odds ratio—is close to the random ROC, only 20% along the way from the random ROC to the ideal point.

the way; a point with odds ratio = 81.0 is *at best* 80% of the way. [Note: How far the peak of the curve is from the random ROC is determined by $(\sqrt{OR} - 1)/(\sqrt{OR} + 1)$, a rescaling of the odds ratio referred to as Yule's Index.] The convergence of all the ROC curves in the corners means that in the two corners of the ROC plane, all those odds ratios may sit near the random ROC regardless of their values. In these corners we can barely distinguish the location of a risk factor with odds ratio = 22 from one with odds ratio = 2.0 or 1.0. Yet with a large enough sample size, risk factors located here may be statistically significant.

In discussing each of the potency measures thus far, we have ignored the diagnosis line and thus the prevalence, *P*. We have not even bothered to put the diagnosis line on Figures 9.5–9.8. Yet when we discussed the harm-to-benefit balance, it was clear that how many people will have the outcome (i.e., the prevalence, *P*) had to be considered to understand the clinical significance of a risk factor. Unfortunately, the risk difference, the risk ratios, and the odds ratio (and all the potency measures that are rescalings of the odds ratio, including the log odds ratio, Yule's index, and gamma) all do not consider *P*.

The Phi Coefficient Does Consider Prevalence but Does Not Consider How Much Those People Will Be Harmed or Benefited

Let us now turn our attention to the *phi coefficient*, a measure of potency that does consider how many people will be harmed or benefited—that is, considers the prevalence, *P*. The most common measure of association between two variables measured on a scale (as opposed to binary variables) is the product moment correlation coefficient. The phi coefficient is the product moment correlation coefficient applied to binary data. The phi coefficient is often used by researchers familiar with the product moment correlation in other contexts, but it is rarely advocated as a potency measure in risk estimation. However, we address it here to illustrate how it includes consideration the prevalence of the outcome (*P*) as well as the level of the risk factor (*Q*).

Remember that to "see" *Q* we draw a line through the risk factor parallel to the diagnosis line that cuts the random ROC at the point (*Q*, *Q*). Then, as shown in Figure 9.9, we draw two nested boxes, both with one corner at the point (*Q*, *Q*). One box (the larger shaded box shown in Figure 9.9) has its other corner at the ideal point. The other box (the smaller box in Figure 9.9) has its other corner at the risk factor (here minority). The ratio of the areas of the smaller box to the bigger box is the square of the phi coefficient [in Figure 9.9, that ratio is 0.19; i.e., the phi coefficient = $PP'(\text{Se} - \text{Sp}')/(PP'QQ')^{1/2} = 0.43$].

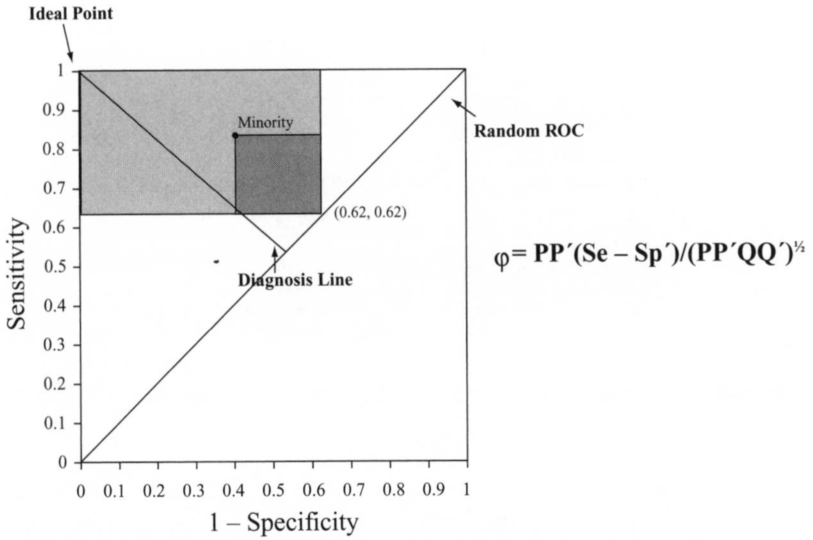

Figure 9.9. How the phi coefficient for the risk factor minority is measured in the ROC plane. The phi coefficient is the ratio of the area of the smaller shaded box to the area of the larger shaded box, where each box has one corner at the point (Q, Q) = (0.62, 0.62). The larger box has its other corner at the ideal point, while the smaller box has its other corner at the location of the risk factor.

If the point determined by the factor lies directly on the random ROC, phi is zero; if it lies near the ideal point, phi is close to one. As the point moves along the line parallel to the diagnosis line from the random ROC to the ideal point, phi moves from zero to some maximal value determined by the relationship of P to Q. For example, in Figure 9.10, we move the point corresponding to the risk factor along the line parallel to the diagnosis line until it hits the upper boundary. This point generates the maximal value phi can reach (0.83) for the risk factor we're considering where $Q = 0.62$ and $P = 0.53$. Only when $P = Q$ can the maximal value of one be achieved. Of special note is the fact that the 2×2 chi square test statistic, the test statistic almost universally used for testing whether there is any association, equals the product of the sample size and the phi coefficient squared. Thus, even though the phi coefficient is almost never used as a measure of potency—that is, as an indicator of clinical significance—the square of phi is almost always used as the indicator of statistical significance.

The phi coefficient has several advantages over the measures of potency we have discussed so far (risk difference, risk ratios, odds ratio). The phi coefficient does consider the prevalence of the outcome (P) in addition to the

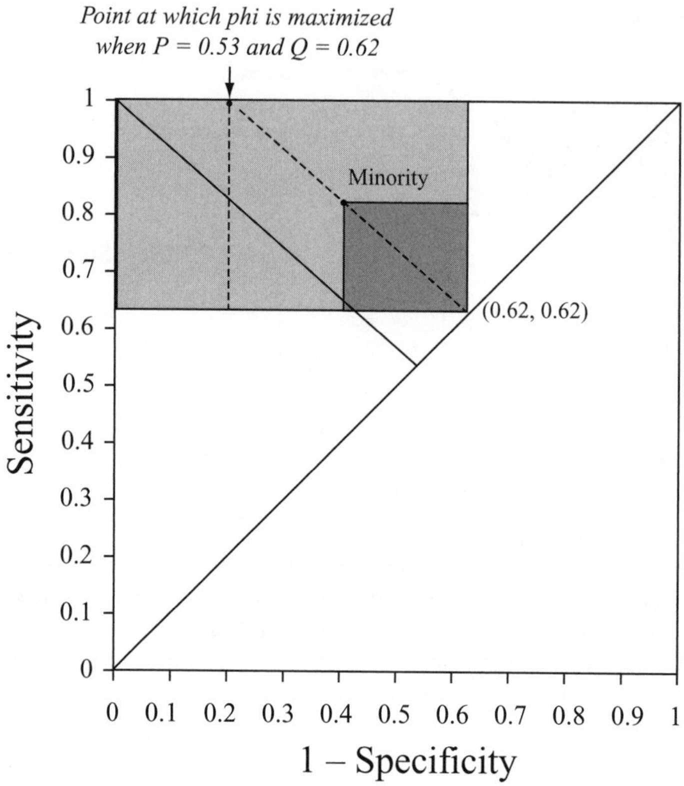

Figure 9.10. How the maximal phi coefficient is determined for given values of P and Q. Only when $P = Q$ can the maximal value of one be achieved, since for perfect prediction the proportion of persons considered high risk by the risk factor (Q) must equal the prevalence of the outcome (P).

sensitivity and specificity—that is, it does consider how many people potentially could be harmed and benefited. It is familiar to those with experience with the product moment correlation coefficient and is closely related to the 2 × 2 chi square test statistic that is almost universally the basis of claims of statistical significance. However, although it does consider the number potentially harmed and benefited, it does *not* acknowledge *how much* potential harm and benefit may occur. That is, the phi coefficient does acknowledge that a particular risk factor potentially could harm, say, 10% of the population and benefit, say, 20%. But what the phi coefficient does not take into account is whether that harm is a minor inconvenience or mild pain or is as significant as disability or death or, likewise, whether that benefit is a minor convenience or mild relief or as significant as avoiding disability or death.

The Weighted Kappa Coefficient Acknowledges Both How Many People Might Be Harmed and Benefited and the Extent of That Harm and Benefit

To introduce the weighted kappa coefficient, let us return to our initial discussion on harm versus benefit from Example 9.1:

EXAMPLE 9.3

As in Example 9.1, suppose researchers have an intervention targeted at preventing schizophrenia. In addition, they have a risk factor to determine who is of high risk for developing schizophrenia and would probably benefit from an intervention. In Example 9.1, we counted how many of those identified by the risk factor would benefit to compare to how many would be harmed, but we did not compare how much harm versus how much benefit occurred, that is, how much harm occurs when an intervention intended to prevent schizophrenia is given to someone who will never develop schizophrenia, and how much benefit occurs when that intervention is given to someone who will develop schizophrenia. Now for this example, let's also consider the degree of harm and benefit by assuming that the benefit of being correctly identified and treated is, on average, \$B, while the harm of being incorrectly identified and unnecessarily treated is, on average, \$H, where \$B and \$H could be zero or could be very large depending on the population, the treatment, and the perceived benefits of preventing schizophrenia. Note that we are only using dollar signs as a reminder that the harm and benefit correspond to costs and benefits. \$B and \$H cannot necessarily be measured or statistically estimated using a monetary scale.

In Example 9.3, as in Example 9.1, the proportion of people in the population who will benefit is $P{\cdot}\mathrm{Se}$, while the proportion of people who will be harmed is $P'{\cdot}\mathrm{Sp}'$. Using these proportions as a starting point, we are going to show how we can derive a measure of potency that includes the proportion benefited and harmed, as well as the extent to which those proportions are benefited and harmed. The measure of potency we are deriving is the weighted kappa coefficient (those wishing to skip the details and take it on trust that this measure does indeed capture these issues may want to skip down to equation 5 below, the equation for the weighted kappa coefficient).

To begin, the overall per-person net benefit is the proportion that will benefit times the benefit (\$B) minus the proportion that will be harmed times the harm (\$H), or per-person net benefit for using a risk factor:

$$P{\cdot}\mathrm{Se}{\cdot}\$\mathrm{B} - P'{\cdot}\mathrm{Sp}'{\cdot}\$\mathrm{H} \tag{1}$$

Now, suppose we were to resort to random decision making. Recall that when we described the random ROC we said that for a decision made randomly (e.g., flipping a coin, tossing a die), the sensitivity equals one minus the specificity, which equals the level (i.e., Se = Sp' = Q—a mathematical demonstration is included in the appendix). Of course, we would want the sensitivity and specificity of the risk factor at least to exceed the sensitivity and specificity of random decision making, so replacing both Se and Sp' by Q, we would want Equation (1) to exceed the per-person net benefit for random decision making:

$$P{\cdot}Q{\cdot}\$\mathrm{B} - P'{\cdot}Q{\cdot}\$\mathrm{H} \tag{2}$$

To see how much better than random we are doing, we simply subtract equation 2 from equation 1 to derive the additional per-person benefit for using a risk factor instead of randomly deciding:

$$P{\cdot}(\mathrm{Se} - Q){\cdot}\$\mathrm{B} - P'{\cdot}(\mathrm{Sp}' - Q){\cdot}\$\mathrm{H} \tag{3}$$

Thus, minimally to have any potency at all, equation 3 would have to be greater than zero. Ideally, we'd want to have perfect sensitivity and specificity (Se = Sp = 1). If we had perfect sensitivity and specificity, equation 3 would become the additional benefit for using a perfect risk factor instead of randomly deciding:

$$P{\cdot}Q'{\cdot}\$\mathrm{B} + P'{\cdot}Q{\cdot}\$\mathrm{H} \tag{4}$$

We can't really expect to achieve perfection, but to see how far between random and perfect we'd come using that risk factor, we'd divide equation 3 by equation 4 and (skipping over some algebra) we'd arrive at what is known as the weighted kappa coefficient, which defines the ratio of the benefit over random of using a risk factor to using a perfect risk factor:

$$\kappa(r) = [P{\cdot}Q'{\cdot}r{\cdot}\kappa(1) + P'{\cdot}Q{\cdot}r'{\cdot}\kappa(0)]/[P{\cdot}Q'{\cdot}r + P'{\cdot}Q{\cdot}r'] \tag{5}$$

where $\kappa(1) = (\mathrm{Se} - Q)/Q'$ and $\kappa(0) = (\mathrm{Sp} - Q')/Q$. Note that we provided a somewhat simpler, but completely equivalent, equation for this kappa coefficient in Table 9.1:

$$\kappa(r) = P{\cdot}P'(\mathrm{Se} - \mathrm{Sp}')/(P{\cdot}Q'{\cdot}r + P'{\cdot}Q{\cdot}r')$$

Here r is an indicator of the benefit to harm balance, selected to best represent the relative harms and benefits of the particular risk factor and outcome of interest:

$$r = \$\mathrm{B}/(\$\mathrm{B} + \$\mathrm{H})$$

with $r' = 1 - r$ or \$H/(\$B + \$H). The value of r ranges from zero to one—where $r = 0$ indicates that the harm done to false positives totally overwhelms the benefit done to true positives and $r = 1$ indicates that the benefit totally overwhelms the harm. When the benefit and harm are roughly equal, or there is neither harm nor benefit (as with the available remedies to the common cold), $r = 0.5$. Note that \$B and \$H are not necessarily measured exactly—they only serve to help to set the value of r that is, by and large, based on subjective judgments by risk evaluators and risk managers. Actually, the exact value of r, in practice, usually matters very little. What typically matters is whether r is nearer to zero, nearer to one-half, or nearer to one.

Let us return to the ROC plane and show, as we have done with the other measures of potency, how the kappa coefficient measures the distance of the risk factor from the random ROC and from the Ideal point. The kappa coefficient uses the same two boxes as did the phi coefficient (see Figure 9.11). However, instead of computing a ratio of areas, $\kappa(1)$ is the ratio of the heights of the two boxes, and $\kappa(0)$ is the ratio of the widths of the two boxes. $\kappa(r)$ is

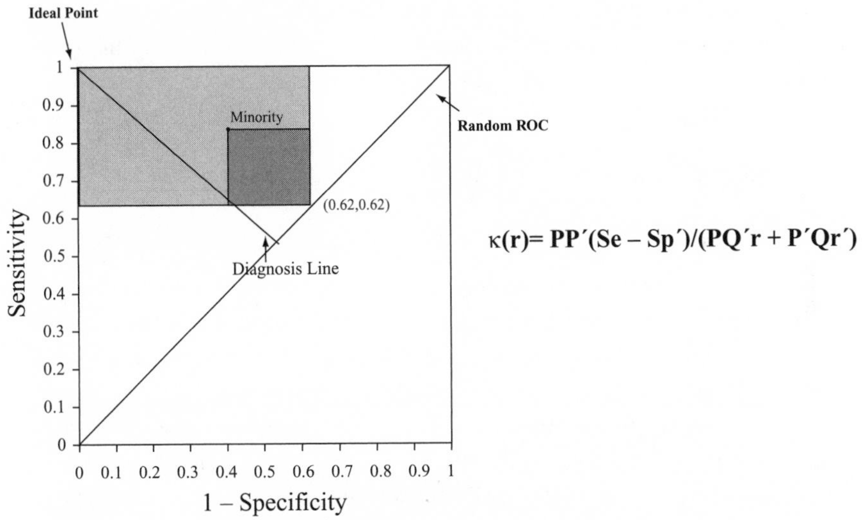

Figure 9.11. How the weighted kappa coefficient for the risk factor minority is measured in the ROC plane. $\kappa(1)$ is the ratio of the height of the smaller box to the height of the larger box, where each box has one corner at the point $(Q, Q) = (0.62, 0.62)$. The larger box has its other corner at the ideal point, while the smaller box has its other corner at the location of the risk factor. $\kappa(0)$ is the ratio of the widths of the two boxes. $\kappa(r)$ is a weighted average of these two ratios.

a weighted average of these two ratios that reflects the relative emphasis put on sensitivity via $\kappa(1)$ and specificity via $\kappa(0)$.

Like every measure of potency, the kappa coefficient also considers the accuracy of the risk factor (sensitivity and specificity). Like the phi coefficient (but not the risk difference, the risk ratios, or the odds ratio), the kappa coefficient considers the relative number of those at risk of benefit and harm (P). But unlike the other potency measures, the kappa coefficient also considers the potential relative degree of benefit versus harm reflected in r. Researchers can select the r that best fits their assessment of the situation to evaluate the potency. For example, researchers would select an $r = 0$ when false positives are overwhelmingly more worrisome than missing a few cases (e.g., for identifying those in need of surgical or radical interventions). Researchers might select an $r = 1$ when identifying as many true positives as possible is the most important consideration even if that means falsely identifying a few (e.g., for mass screening where each positive identification would be checked by a doctor). Finally a researcher might select $r = 0.5$ if the risk factors were only being evaluated for scientific interest and no intervention is contemplated, or if the harms and benefits tend to balance out.

Surprisingly enough, almost all of the potency measures we have already discussed are actually closely related to some kappa coefficient, although some require rescaling to see the relationship. That is, each is related to a kappa coefficient with some particular value of r. For example, the risk difference always equals $\kappa(P')$. Both risk ratios rescaled are also closely related to two different kappas:

$$(\mathrm{RR}_1 - 1)/[\mathrm{RR}_1 + (P'/P)] = \kappa(0)$$

$$(\mathrm{RR}_2 - 1)/[\mathrm{RR}_2 + (P/P')] = \kappa(1)$$

The phi coefficient is the geometric mean of the two extreme kappas: $[\kappa(0) \cdot \kappa(1)]^{1/2}$. A potency measure we have not discussed that is often seen in risk research, the attributable risk, is simply $\kappa(0)$. Without meaning to, risk researchers have come up with different measures of potency that are actually just different ways of weighting the sensitivity and specificity, thus corresponding to one or another kappa coefficient. The one measure of potency that doesn't fit this pattern is the odds ratio, unfortunately the most commonly used one.

Recall that one of our major objections to the odds ratio, the risk difference, and the risk ratio is that their values are very difficult to interpret when the plotted risk factor lies in either the lower right corner or the upper left corner of the ROC plane. This problem is solved by the kappa coefficient. For example, selecting an r close to zero indicates that the researcher believes specificity is the most important consideration. Then a point in the lower left corner (where the specificity is near one) may indeed be a better choice than one closer to the center or in the upper right corner, even if it does appear to be closer to the random ROC. For example, if we use $\kappa(0)$ to evaluate the three IHDP risk factors we've been considering for low IQ among premature low-birth-weight children, Hispanic is the most potent [$\kappa(0) = 0.44$ for Hispanic, 0.35 for minority, and 0.33 for black]. Similarly selecting an *r* close to one indicates that the researcher believes sensitivity is the most important consideration, in which case a point in the upper right corner (where the sensitivity is near 1) may indeed be a better choice than one closer to the center or in the lower left corner. Then, if we use $\kappa(1)$, minority is the most potent risk factor [$\kappa(1) = 0.54$ for minority, 0.06 for Hispanic, and 0.31 for black]. The challenge, then, is to pick an appropriate value of *r* and evaluate the risk factor accordingly.

How Do Researchers Select the Optimal Harm-to-Benefit Balance (*r*)?

Let's return to the IHDP example and now recall why we are looking at these different risk factors for low IQ among children who were born prematurely with a low birth weight. The objective was to identify risk factors at birth for low IQ and thus to identify those most in need of early intervention to increase school readiness. A lot of considerations need to go into selecting an optimal *r* for this situation. On the benefit side, how much do researchers think they can improve IQ if they correctly identified the high-risk children early? What are the benefits to increasing IQ? Would improvement in IQ really translate to improvement in school readiness? If it did, what would the benefits be of increasing school readiness (e.g., improvement in their quality of life, society savings in terms of having to provide programs for children who are not ready for public school)? On the harm side, would researchers harm these children or their families by labeling them high risk? Could the proposed intervention adversely affect a child or the family? How expensive is the intervention? Who is going to pay for the intervention, the family or society?

Some risk researchers may ask, Why is it the responsibility of risk researchers to pay any attention at all to such benefits and harm? Isn't that the responsibility of medical decision makers? Risk researchers shouldn't even pretend to have the expertise to make such judgments and typically don't have the motivation to take on such responsibility. The fundamental issue is not to place a responsibility on the shoulders of risk researchers that indeed properly belongs to medical decision makers, but rather to assure that that risk researchers do not mislead medical decision makers by reporting results that are incorrect, misleading, or easily misinterpreted. Thus, risk researchers cannot ignore the problem. However, there are a few shortcuts that might help researchers to decide what to report.

Although we keep talking about $\kappa(0)$ and $\kappa(1)$, there are very few risk factors that correspond either to no benefit at all or to no harm at all. Generally, there is at least some benefit to identifying a true positive and at least some harm to identifying a false positive. Frequently, after long and intense discussion of all the possible sources of benefit and harm, researchers will come to the conclusion that the benefits and harms tend to balance out, and choose $r = 0.5$. When researchers use a weighted kappa, they typically use $\kappa(0.5)$, commonly called Cohen's kappa. Thus, one strategy is to set r equal to 0.5, unless there is strong reason indicating otherwise.

Another tactic is based on a completely different approach. Consider these three questions:

1. Of N individuals labeled high risk, how many will get the disorder? *Answer:* $N \cdot A/Q$, or $N \cdot \text{PVP}$.
2. Of N individuals labeled low risk, how many will get the disorder? *Answer:* $N \cdot B/Q'$, or $N \cdot \text{PVN}'$.
3. How many individuals in each risk group would we have had to sample to have one more case in the high-risk group than in the low-risk group? *Answer:* $N \cdot \text{PVP} = N \cdot \text{PVN}' + 1$, or $N = 1/(\text{PVP} - \text{PVN}')$

We can show that the value $1/(\text{PVP} - \text{PVN}')$ is the same as $1/\kappa(Q)$. Thus, we can set $r = Q$, and use that to compute the weighted kappa. The result is number needed to treat/take (NNT), the measure we recommended in Chapter 4 as an easy-to-interpret shortcut. Rescaled NNT corresponds to one form of weighted kappa, where the weight is determined by Q, the proportion of the population to be considered high risk.

While the debate goes on, a good solution would be to report P and both $\kappa(0)$ and $\kappa(1)$ in addition to whichever measure of potency is preferred, in which case any medical decision maker, researcher, or savvy medical consumer can use their own value of r to evaluate the potency of the risk factor from their own point of view. (Equations to reconstruct the 2×2 contingency table—and thus any measure of potency—from P, $\kappa(0)$, and $\kappa(1)$ are included in the mathematical demonstrations in the appendix.)

Researchers Can Also Use the ROC to Compare the Potencies of Multiple Risk Factors

While we have shown that we can use the ROC to visualize the different measures of potency, we still have not discussed how we use the ROC to compare the potency of different risk factors for a single outcome in a single population. Using the risk factors identified in the IHDP control group for low IQ, let's return to visually evaluating those risk factors in the ROC plane. In our earlier discussion, we included three race/ethnicity risk factors—any of which might be considered too controversial to actually use to target an intervention. Imagine the controversy, if, for example, policy makers decided to provide high-quality day care to black or Hispanic premature low-birth-weight children for the purposes of improving IQ. That not only would smack of some sort of infant affirmative action but also might even be considered labeling and thus discriminatory. Thus, let's expand our sights a little and consider two other potential risk factors considered in this study: maternal education at the time of birth and birth weight. The neonatologists and pediatricians involved in the design of the IHDP study were quite certain that birth weight (or the highly correlated gestational age) would be major predictors of low IQ.

Maternal education and birth weight are not binary measures—maternal education was measured on a five-point scale, while weight was measured in grams. However, we can dichotomize each of these risk factors in a variety of ways using different cut points and consider the potency of each different dichotomization. For example, we can consider as high risk those children whose mothers had less than an eighth grade education ("never attended high school") and those children whose mothers had more than an eighth grade education as low risk. Alternatively, we can consider as high risk those children whose mothers had less than a high school diploma ("not high school grad"), or those whose mother never attended college ("never attended college"), or those whose mothers did not graduate from college ("not college grad"). We could dichotomize birth weight at 100 gram increments from less than 900 grams up to less than 2,400 grams. All of these risk factors are plotted in Figure 9.12.

After locating all the risk factors, we draw the upper boundary of all these points by connecting all the points on the outer edge and the two corner points with straight lines (the "convex hull" of these points—see Figure 9.12). What results is a "curve" called the *ROC curve* related to this family of risk factors. All points below the ROC curve can now be set aside from consideration, since, for each of these, there is a point on the ROC curve that has *both* better sensitivity and better specificity. [Note: such a point may be a combination of two risk factors currently under consideration.]

Here we see the surprising result that birth weight has very little potency for detecting those who will have low IQ, because all the points related to dichotomizations of birth weight (the dashes) are barely above the random ROC and far below the ROC curve. Thus, the risk factors that determine

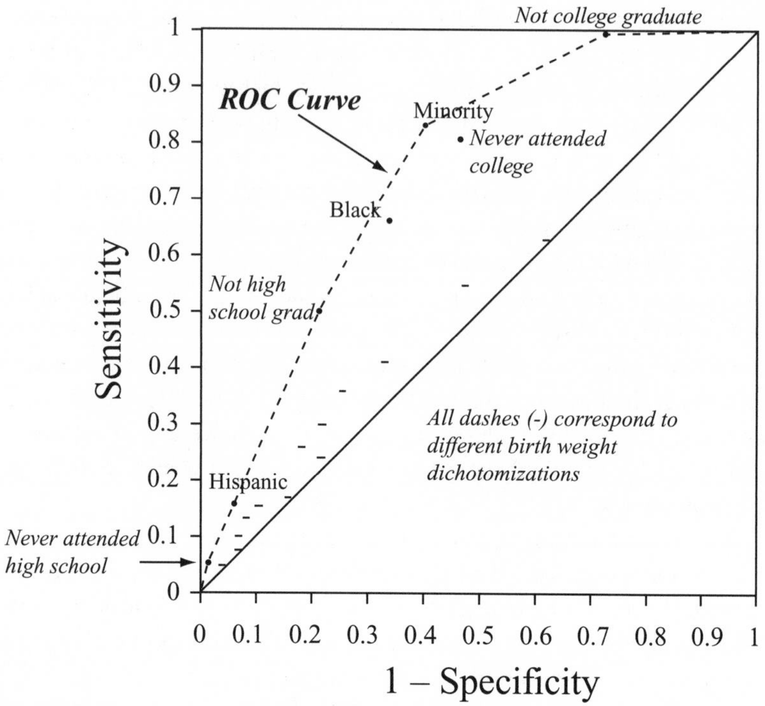

Figure 9.12. The ROC plane with many plotted risk factors for low IQ in this population of low-birth-weight premature children. The ROC curve is the upper boundary of all the points connecting all the points and the two corners of the random ROC. Points along the ROC curve are the most potent; risk factors located below the curve have either lower sensitivity and/or lower specificity than risk factors (or combinations of risk factors) located on the curve.

points on the ROC curve are the maternal education factor with three cut points, minority, and Hispanic. Note also that if the ethnicity/race risk factors were removed from consideration, the ROC curve would be totally determined by maternal education.

Now, to select which of these five risk factors located on the ROC curve is the best, we need to select a value of *r* and then compute κ(r) for each point on the ROC curve, selecting the one with the highest value for κ(r).

For example, here if *r* is 0.5 (about equal harm and benefit), the optimal choice would be to treat all minorities, that is, treat *Q* = 62% of this low-birth-weight premature population. Of those treated, 70% (PVP) would have gone on to have low IQ in absence of intervention, whereas of those not treated (1 – PVN) only 25% will go on to have low IQ. If, on the other hand, we removed race/ethnicity from the list, the optimal choice would be to treat all those whose mothers were not high school graduates ($Q = 37\%$). Then, of those treated, 72% (PVP) would have gone on to have low IQ in absence of intervention, whereas of those not treated (1 – PVN), 42% will go on to have low IQ. The optimal decisions for other values of *r* are set out in Table 9.2, as well as the comparisons with no intervention and universal intervention.

As you can see in Table 9.2, the higher the benefit and the lower the cost, the larger the proportion of the population that should be treated—that is, as *r* increases, the percentage to treat (Q) also increases. Also, if we compare these optimal decisions to no intervention ($Q = 0\%$) and universal intervention ($Q = 100\%$), we see that the lower the *r*, the closer we come to recommending doing nothing; the higher the *r*, the closer we come to recommending universal intervention.

Moreover, the percentage of people who really may benefit from treatment among those who are considered high risk (PVP) increases as *r* decreases. That is, as *r* moves toward zero, the more harm outweighs benefit and the more likely we would be to recommend treating fewer people (Q is decreasing), but a higher percentage of them would be the actual people who would benefit from treatment.

At the same time, as *r* moves toward zero, a higher percentage of those who would not be recommended for treatment would have that outcome—that is, they might have benefited from the intervention had they gotten it. Since then treatment could reduce risk only for those treated, we would expect that the reduction in risk in the total population would be least when *r* is close to zero and greatest when *r* is close to one. In the extreme, if we decided to treat no one, the risk in the population of 53% would remain 53%. At the other extreme, with universal prevention, how much the risk would be reduced would depend on the effectiveness of the treatment offered.

Finally, if for whatever reason it was decided that ethnicity/race could not be used to identify high-risk subjects, "Not high school grad" would replace minority as optimal for *r* between 0.2 and 0.8, and there would be some loss, but not much.

So after all this discussion of potency measures, why draw the ROC plane when we still used a summary measure of potency to describe potency and to select the optimal risk factor? The answer is: we did not have to. Had we calculated the kappa coefficient, using an appropriate value for *r* for all of the risk factors under consideration, we would have arrived at the same answer. What the curve bought us is the opportunity to visualize how the various risk factors performed both individually and in relation to each other—a feat that is difficult to comprehend by just looking at a set of numbers. The ROC plot allowed us to see surprising results such as that birth weight—implicated in the past as being a strong indicator of poor IQ—was here at best a weak risk

Table 9.2
The Most Optimal Risk Factor for Different Values of *r*

r	Who to Treat?	% to Treat (*Q*)	% Who Would Have Low IQ If Not Treated (PVP)	% Those Not Treated Who Will Have Low IQ (1 – PVN)
None	None	0%	N/A: no one treated	53%
0	Never attended high school	3%	77%	53%
0.1	Not high school graduate	37%	72%	42%
0.2–0.8	Minority	62%	70%	25%
0 9–1.0	Not college graduate	86%	61%	6%
Universal	All	100%	53%	N/A: everyone treated

factor (perhaps because the population was limited to low-birth-weight children). These results suggest that much of the reason for low IQ in this population does not appear to be biological (related to birth weight, prematurity, or birth complications) but is related to socioeconomic class. What the ROC plane gives us is a way to visually process a lot of important information about each risk factor and to visually comprehend why we do or do not advocate use of some of the commonly used measures of potency.

Conclusion and Summary

We've repeated it many times: statistical significance is simply not enough. When researchers move beyond statistical significance and recognize the need to acknowledge both the possible benefits and the possible harm from using a risk factor, they will be motivated to present a measure of potency that communicates both. Many commonly reported measures, notably the odds ratio, fail to explicitly take into account the benefits and harm of true and false identification. We propose that the measure of potency that best communicates both is the weighted kappa coefficient, with the weight reflecting the relative balance of harm to false positives versus benefit to true positives. However, recognizing the challenges in "throwing away" whichever potency measure researchers are most familiar with, we would suggest they also report P, $\kappa(0)$, and $\kappa(1)$, from which a little effort would yield any other measure of association.

However, researchers' goals should not be to find the one and only best risk factor. If it were, we would rarely have good prediction since typically each individual risk factor does not, by itself, present very high potency. Instead, what researchers are seeking is to know how multiple risk factors work together to produce an outcome. Thus, in Chapter 10 we describe the technical details for identifying mediators, moderators, proxy, overlapping, and independent risk factors. Chapter 11, the final chapter in Part III, then builds from how risk factors work together to how researchers can use multiple risk factors to best predict who is of highest and lowest risk of the outcome.

- Determining the clinical significance of risk factors is a complex process that should include consideration of the benefit of correctly identifying those who will have the outcome (true positives) and the harm of incorrectly identifying those who will not have the outcome (false positives).
- In a particular population, sensitivity is the probability that someone who will have the outcome is classified as high risk. Sensitivity

measures the probability that someone who will have the outcome will be correctly identified (a true positive).

- In a particular population, specificity is the probability that someone who will not have the outcome is classified as low risk. Specificity measures the probability someone who will not have the outcome will be correctly identified (a true negative). One minus specificity measures the probability that someone who will not have the outcome will be incorrectly identified (a false positive).
- In the ROC approach to evaluate potency, we plot the sensitivity of a risk factor against one minus the specificity.
- The ROC plane has two main "landmarks": the random ROC and the ideal point. The random ROC is a line connecting the lower left corner of the plot to the upper right corner. This line represents all points where sensitivity equals one minus specificity equals the "level" of the factor. All factors located on this line cannot be risk factors; rather, they are factors that are randomly associated with the outcome (see Figure 9.1).
- The ideal point is located in the upper left corner of the plot. At this point the sensitivity and specificity of the risk factor are both one, corresponding to the location of a risk factor that perfectly predicts the outcome (see Figure 9.1).
- The diagnosis line in the ROC plane connects the ideal point with the point (P, P) on the random ROC. All risk factors lie on a lie parallel to the diagnosis line and cross the random ROC at the point (Q, Q). The diagnosis line is critical to being able to "read off" P and Q from the ROC plot and use them with the sensitivity and specificity to determine the proportion of the population harmed and benefited by using a risk factor to predict an outcome.
- All measures of potency are different ways of measuring how much better than random (i.e., distance from the random ROC) and/or how much worse than perfect (i.e., distance from the ideal point) a risk factor performs.
- By looking at how different potency measures measure the distances from the plotted risk factor to the random ROC and/or to the ideal point, we can point out some of the problems with some of the more common potency measures. For example, the risk difference favors risk factors with levels close to 0.5, regardless of what the prevalence of the outcome of interest. The risk ratios can provide completely opposite indications of the potency of the risk factor, raising the issue of which one is correct and which one should be used. The odds ratio can indicate strong potency for many risk factors very close to the

random ROC. In addition, the odds ratio cannot differentiate the potency of risk factors with levels either close to zero or close to one. None of these measures considers the prevalence of the outcome in question (*P*), and thus they do not consider how many people may potentially be harmed and how many may potentially be benefited.

- The prevalence of the outcome (*P*) is considered in calculating the value of the phi coefficient. The phi coefficient is closely related to the commonly used 2 × 2 chi square statistic but is rarely used in risk research. The phi coefficient does not, however, include consideration of how much harm or benefit may occur.
- We recommend use of the kappa coefficient because it does consider how many people are harmed or benefited by using a risk factor to predict an outcome, as well as how much harm and benefit may occur. The kappa coefficient uses a parameter *r* that estimates the relative weight of harm to false positives and benefits to true positives.
- Typically, the actual value of r does not matter as much as whether or not it is closer to zero, closer to one, or closer to 0.5. Some shortcuts researchers can take is to report Cohen's kappa (where r = 0.5), report the NNT [$1/\kappa(Q)$], or report *P*, $\kappa(0)$, and $\kappa(1)$ to allow any medical decision maker, researcher, or savvy medical consumer to evaluate the potency of the risk factor with their own value of r.
- To use the ROC approach to select the most potent of a set of risk factors, we plot all of the risk factors and connect the outermost points together. The line segments that connect the outmost points (the "convex hull") are called the ROC curve. All points below the ROC curve should be removed from consideration because they are less potent than either the points on the ROC curve or some combination of the points on the ROC curve. Then, selecting which of the risk factors located on the ROC curve is a matter of determining an appropriate r and calculating the kappa coefficient for each of these points (see Figure 9.12).
- Drawing an ROC plot when evaluating the potency of risk factors is actually not necessary. Since ultimately we used a kappa coefficient to evaluate points on the ROC curve, we could have calculated the kappa coefficient for all points and selected the biggest one. However, the ROC curve allow us to visually process a lot of important information about each risk factor and possibly gain insights into particular risk factors that we may not have otherwise understood.

10

How Do We Do a Moderator–Mediator Analysis?

A tale of two gold prospectors: Both select an area where they suspect there is gold. Both begin with the same equipment and motivation, and both start the same way. They dredge up a likely sample to begin to pan for gold. Now their paths separate.

The first prospector examines his pan carefully, setting aside all the rocks and pebbles. Then, he begins carefully to wash away the sand and silt. He sets all this debris aside. He examines anything in the pan likely to be a flake or nugget of gold and, if not gold, sets that aside. As much as he is able, he tries to clump flakes into tiny nuggets and tiny nuggets into larger ones. At the end of the day, he will carry his collection to the assayers to find out the value of what he has found.

The second prospector is very reluctant to set anything aside. After all, he reasons, what may look like rocks, pebbles, sand, and silt may in fact hide gold. Of course, he may be right, so he piles more and more samples into his pans. At the end of the day, he certainly has a lot of samples!

This story is a parable for the problems faced by risk researchers. True causal factors, the "gold" of risk research, are buried in a mass of correlates that are not even risk factors and risk factors that are not causal. Yet risk research has a tradition of simply piling up those correlates and risk factors, much like the second prospector, counting them up or scoring them. How often have you seen checklists in the media asking how many signs and symptoms on a list you have and informing you that, if you've crossed some cut point of check marks, you are at risk of some outcome you'd as soon avoid? For a more formal example, consider the Framingham Index that uses a list of risk factors to compute a score that predicts an individual's risk of heart disease.[1]

Instead, we propose to follow the lead of the first prospector. Is it possible that by doing so, we might set aside and miss a flake or nugget or two? Of course, but that is why we *set aside* rather than discard. While the second prospector probably cannot save the piles of silt and sand forever in hopes that later with better equipment he can dig out more gold, saving data and ideas with modern computers is not an issue. Researchers can always go back and reexamine any materials set aside if there are any doubts.

In Chapter 9 we concluded by noting that individual risk factors often, by themselves, don't do enough in predicting an outcome. We urge that researchers consider multiple risk factors to best understand who will and will not have an outcome. However, our gold prospecting parable illustrates how considering too many risk factors without considering how they fit together may further confuse the prediction of who will and will not have an outcome. In this chapter, we expand the discussion introduced in Chapter 5 on how risk factors work together by describing how researchers can pare down a long list of risk factors to an organized list of few. The goal of doing so is to get to the most important risk factors in identifying causal pathways: moderators and mediators. Here we will review the definitions of the five main "inter-actions," proxy, overlapping, moderator, mediator, and independent, focusing more on the operational definitions we skimmed over in Chapter 5. Then we will present a step-by-step guide of how to identify these inter-actions (i.e., do a "moderator–mediator analysis") among a set of identified risk factors.

Before Doing a Moderator–Mediator Analysis, Researchers Must First Identify the True Risk Factors

Before we step through a moderator–mediator analysis, let's review what comes before: identifying which potential risk factors are indeed risk factors. Part II addressed issues of research design—a topic we do not intend to revisit in this chapter. However, first and foremost, we do not want to discount the vital design issues that come into play long before a moderator–mediator analysis proceeds. Specifically, to be able to identify risk factors—at least those that are not fixed at birth—the data need to come from a well-designed, longitudinal study.

The first step in the analysis of such a longitudinal study is to evaluate every factor that precedes the outcome and set aside those that cannot be shown to have a statistically significant relationship with the outcome. Risk researchers are typically dismayed at how many factors will be set aside at this point. Sometimes researchers will start with 100 or more potential risk factors and rapidly reduce the pool to 5 or 10. But that shouldn't be surprising, because correlates previously identified in cross-sectional studies are very much at risk of being removed as possible risk factors when the requirement of temporal precedence is imposed in a longitudinal study. In addition, factors suggested as risk factors in previous case-control studies often have sampling and measurement biases that result in their not panning out when an appropriate sample is collected and retrospective recall is avoided. As did our gold prospector, researchers must set aside the rocks, pebbles, dirt, and silt in order to have a better chance at the gold.

While trying to get to that gold, however, researchers should not forget to look in the obvious places. Specifically, it is easy to overlook simple risk factors such as age and gender because they are often risk factors for many disorders. However, they are often very important moderators whose omission may steer the research in the wrong direction.

Clearly, if the sample size is small, some true risk factors may be lost simply because the sample size is too small to detect any relationship to the outcome (inadequate power). Perhaps not as obvious, true risk factors that are measured badly, with poor validity and/or poor reliability, are also likely to be lost.

How exactly do we decide which factors should be set aside because their relationship with the outcome is not statistically significant? Almost universally, if the factor is binary (male/female, minority/majority, smoker/nonsmoker), researchers will use a 2×2 chi square test to determine statistical significance. If the risk factor is ordinal, researchers will use a Mann-Whitney or a two-sample *t*-test. We favor the Mann-Whitney test because it involves fewer restrictive assumptions. These tests all test the null hypothesis that the relationship is random.

Before conducting these tests, researchers need to select a significance level. Tests with *p*-values below this chosen significance level will be considered "statistically significant." Some risk researchers will choose to use a 5% significance level for each test, and others will choose to use a more stringent test (e.g., 1% or 0.1%). Since we are usually indulging in multiple testing here, we need to be cautious about false detection of a risk factor. Specifically, if 5% is the chosen significance level, we would expect that if all independent factors proposed were randomly associated with the outcome, 5% would still turn up "statistically significant" and be incorrectly labeled as risk factors.

The choice of a more stringent significance level reflects concern about such proliferation of falsely labeled risk factors, and we would recommend 1% or even 0.1%.

Throughout this chapter, we will use the data from the control group in the Infant Health and Development Program (IHDP)[2] to illustrate each of the steps of a moderator–mediator analysis. We introduced the IHDP data in Chapter 3. In Chapter 9, we evaluated the potency of several potential risk factors for the outcome of low IQ at age three among low-birth-weight, premature children, including black (yes/no), Hispanic (yes/no), minority (yes/no), maternal education (five point scale with four possible cut points), and birth weight (grams, with various possible cut points). Now we add a measure of birth complications called Neonatal Health Index, or NHI.[3] An NHI score of 100 indicates that the birth complications were typical of an infant with that birth weight. The higher the score, the fewer the complications; the lower the score, the more serious the complications relative to other infants with the same birth weight. (This scale is similar to that used for IQ testing.) We also add the Bayley Mental Development Index (MDI12) and the Bayley Motor Development Index (PDI12) obtained by testing the infants at 12 months of (corrected) age, also measured on an IQ-like scale. [Note: There are more potential risk factors we could consider, such as site and gender. For purposes of this demonstration, however, we are limiting consideration to these eight potential risk factors.]

To determine which of these eight potential risk factors are true risk factors, we calculate the Spearman rank correlation coefficient between each of the factors and the outcome, and a *p*-value, which if "small," indicates the correlation is statistically significantly different than zero. These correlation coefficients and *p*-values are shown in Table 10.1. The correlation coefficient provides a crude indicator of the strength of the relationship between the factor and the outcome (i.e., the potency). Because we have selected a Spearman rank correlation coefficient, instead of the more common Pearson correlation coefficient that assumes the original data have a bivariate normal distribution, the *p*-values indicating whether or not the correlation is significantly different than zero are equivalent to the tests we recommended earlier (the 2×2 chi square test for a binary risk factor and a Mann-Whitney test for an ordinal risk factor) for determining which potential risk factors are true risk factors.

Thus, as shown in Table 10.1, neither NHI nor birth weight can be shown to be a risk factor for low IQ in this population because their *p*-values are larger than our chosen significance level of 0.01. (Remember, this population consists of low-birth-weight children in the first place, and this may not be true in other populations.) We saw this same result when we noted in

Table 10.1
The Correlations of Eight Potential Risk Factors for the Outcome of Low IQ

Potential Risk Factor	Spearman Correlation	*p*-Value
NHI	–0.048	0.276
Birth weight	–0.060	0.173
Mother's education	–0.403	0.001
Black	0.323	0.001
Hispanic	0.151	0.001
Minority	0.433	0.001
Bayley Mental Development Index (MDI12)	–0.402	0.001
Bayley Motor Development Index (PDI12)	–0.231	0.001

Chapter 9 that different dichotomizations of birth weight plotted in the ROC plane were very close to the random ROC.

On the other hand, we have six bona fide risk factors for low IQ at age three among low-birth-weight-premature children (mother's education, black, Hispanic, minority, MDI12, and PDI12), as their *p*-values are smaller than 0.01 (all <.001). Just looking at these six, we realize that there are probably redundancies (e.g., three different indicators of race) and various relationships (e.g., level of education and race—both related to socioeconomic status) that potentially could confuse how someone might use these risk factors to both estimate the risk of low IQ and hypothesize an intervention to prevent it.

The remainder of this chapter we devote to describing how we can begin to understand and identify these interrelationships by using the six risk factors we have just identified in the IHDP data and by following the steps we conceptually described in Chapter 5:

1. Sort the multiple risk factors by time.
2. For all the risk factors in each time slot, identify and combine overlapping risk factors and set aside proxy risk factors. This leaves only independent risk factors within a time slot. [Note: Usually within each time slot, it does not matter if proxy risk factors or overlapping risk factors are identified first.]
3. For all the now remaining risk factors, examine the relationships between earlier risk factors and later ones. If further proxies are found, set these aside.
4. If a moderator is found, split the population on the moderator and begin the analysis anew within each subgroup defined by the moderator.

5. Finally, for all the now remaining risk factors and possibly within moderator subgroups, examine the relationships between earlier risk factors and later ones to identify mediators.

The First Step Is to Sort the Risk Factors by Time

Temporal precedence is vital in determining how risk factors "work together." In particular, a true causal chain will consist of risk factors that temporally follow one another. For example, if we were to trace how an individual might have contracted AIDS, we might see that having an HIV-infected partner preceded having unprotected sex with that partner, which preceded an HIV infection that preceded the onset of AIDS.

In the IHDP, researchers assessed potential risk factors at birth and every four months following birth until the age of two and evaluated each child at age three for the outcome of low IQ. This repeated assessment simplifies the process of time ordering the potential risk factors during the first three years of life. However, for this demonstration, we will use only a few factors evaluated at birth and at one year of age. When we organize these few risk factors according to temporal precedence (shown in Figure 10.1), we get ethnicity (determined at the time of conception), maternal education at the time of birth, and the two Bayley indices at one year.

In addition to time order, how risk factors "work together" also depends on the correlations among risk factors. Thus, before we begin identifying the interactions, we need a Spearman rank correlation matrix (Table 10.2) between all pairs of potential risk factors under consideration. In Table 10.2, asterisks denote any statistically significant ($p < 0.01$) correlations greater than 0.15 ($r > 0.15$). [Note: We continue to use the Spearman rank correlation coefficient rather than the Pearson correlation coefficient to avoid worries about the limiting assumptions of the Pearson.]

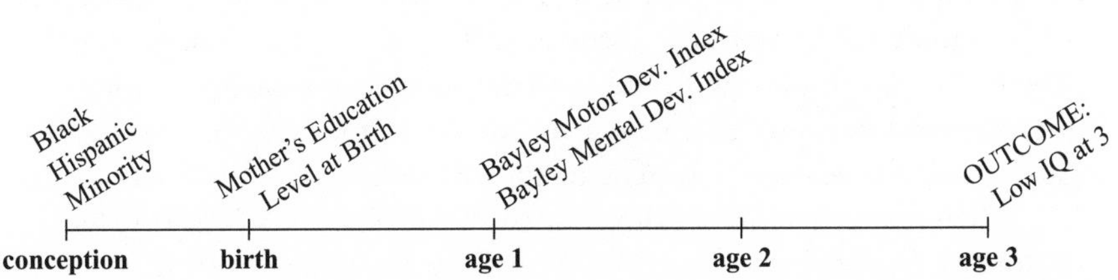

Figure 10.1. The time order of risk factors for low IQ at age three (IHDP control group).

Table 10.2
Correlations among the Six Factors for the Outcome Low IQ

	Black	Hispanic	Minority	MDI12	PDI12
Mother's education	–0.271* ($p < 0.001$)	–0.146 ($p = .001$)	–0.376* ($p < .001$)	0.171* ($p < 0.001$)	0.065 ($p = 0.145$)
Black		–0.367* ($p < .001$)	0.793* ($p < 0.001$)	–0.117 ($p = 0.008$)	0.093 ($p = 0.036$)
Hispanic			0.276* ($p < 0.001$)	–0.074 ($p = 0.094$)	–0.022 ($p = 0.624$)
Minority				–0.170* ($p < 0.001$)	0.082 ($p = 0.065$)
MDI12					0.472* ($p < .001$)

*Statistical significance at the 0.01 level with $r > 0.15$.

Now, armed with both the time precedence (Figure 10.1) and the correlations among risk factors (Table 10.2), we are ready to begin "washing away the sand and silt and setting the debris aside."

Next, Combine Overlapping Risk Factors within Each Time Period

Sometimes when factors of particular interest cannot be measured well, they are measured poorly but repeatedly in different ways. Thus, for example, if researchers do not have a measure of "adequate diet" available, they might measure the number of calories per day or the percentage of those calories from protein, carbohydrates, saturated fat, unsaturated fat, and fiber. In fact, they might even measure each of these in several different ways: by self-report or by informant report, using one-day recall, using seven-day recall, or using diet diaries. What they get is a proliferation of correlated measures, many with poor reliability, producing inconsistent results, but all related to the same underlying construct: "adequate diet." In fact, some or many of these may not be statistically significantly correlated with the outcome of interest, not necessarily because "adequate diet" is not a risk factor, but because the measures don't measure "adequate diet" well enough.

When researchers are seeking "overlapping risk factors," they are looking for risk factors that measure the same thing. Recalling our road analogy, overlapping risk factors are either one road with multiple names or different lanes of the same road. Operationally, two risk factors are overlapping if they are correlated and one does not precede the other, and when used simultaneously, both are important in predicting the outcome. In Figure 10.2, we add to the illustration of different lanes of the same road of Figure 5.2, a depiction of the operational definition. In Figure 10.2, we show two risk factors, labeled X and Y, their time precedence (indicated by left-to-right positioning—in this case we depict no time precedence by placing X or Y equidistant to the outcome, O), and correlation among X and Y and the outcome (O). As we reintroduce each inter-action, we will here include similar depictions of the operational definition. In addition, in the chapter summary below, we have included a diagram that pulls together and summarizes the operational definitions of, and appropriate actions for, all five inter-actions.

In the IHDP example, of the four time points (conception, birth, one year, and three years of age), only two have multiple risk factors (conception and one year of age). Since overlapping risk factors have no time precedence, only the multiple risk factors at the same time point are candidates. Thus, we only consider the three ethnicity measures at birth, and the two Bayley indices at one year of age.

The correlation between the two Bayley indices is high, $r = 0.472$ ($p < 0.001$). We next need to check how the two indices simultaneously predict the outcome. We have many choices of ways to do this, but the most common is to use a logistic regression analysis (LRA), as we will do here. We will

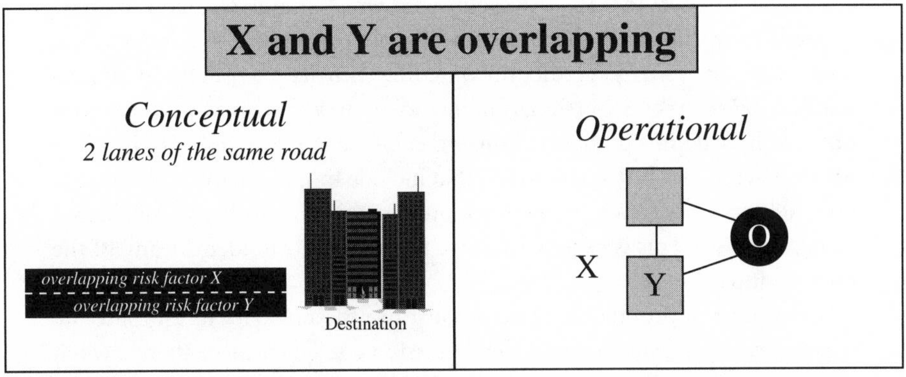

Figure 10.2. An illustration of the conceptual and operational definition of overlapping risk factors. The conceptual illustration shows how overlapping risk factors are like one road with two names or two lanes of the same road. The operational illustration depicts X and Y as risk factors and O as the outcome. Left-to-right positioning of X and Y indicates temporal order (here none). Solid lines between X, Y, and O indicate correlation (here X and Y are correlated and are each correlated with the outcome).

use low IQ as the dependent measure, and the two indices with their interaction as independent measures (here we mean the typical connotation of statistical interaction—not "inter-action").

The basic assumption of an LRA is that the "log odds" of an event is a linear function of whatever is used to predict that event. The *odds* of an event is the ratio of the probability that the event happens to the probability that it does not happen. Thus, for example, if the probability of an event is 0.6, the odds of that event is 0.6/0.4 = 1.5, or as the horse race aficionados would say, 1.5 to 1. What is used in the LRA is the natural logarithm of an odds (log odds, or LO). Thus, if the odds of the event is 1.5, the LO of that event is ln(1.5) = 0.405. The equation of such a model is listed below. B_0 is called the intercept, and although it is important for the calculation, it is not an important consideration for determining inter-actions. The coefficients B_1, B_2, and B_3 are called the regression coefficients, with B_1 and B_2 being referred to "main effects" (since they're each associated with one risk factor) and B_3 being referred to as an "interaction effect" (since it's associated with multiple risk factors). What we are looking at is whether or not each of the main or interaction effects is significantly different than zero (for linguistic simplicity, from here on we are going to say "nonzero" to mean statistically significantly different than zero and place asterisks next to coefficients that are nonzero).

$$\text{LO(Low IQ)} = B_0 + B_1 \cdot \text{MDI12}_C + B_2 \cdot \text{PDI12}_C + B_3 \cdot \text{MDI12}_C \cdot \text{PDI12}_C$$

When one of the coefficients is *not* significantly different from zero, we are unable to assert that the risk factor with which it is associated is helping to predict the outcome. Thus, since we are only looking at risk factors (i.e., those that, taken singly, predict the outcome with accuracy better than random), a logistic regression equation including only that risk factor as a predictor will by definition have a nonzero coefficient associated with it. What we see when we look at such models that include more than one risk factor is how well one risk factor predicts the outcome when another is considered simultaneously. This is exactly what we need to know to identify any of the inter-actions.

However, a problem arises if we just use the raw data to estimate the regression coefficients, because the regression coefficients can change when the coding of the risk factors changes. That is, how researchers numerically represent a measure (e.g., one for being minority, zero for not) affects the values of the regression coefficients. Whether or not a regression coefficient is nonzero (our main interest here), however, does not change with different coding of the data when only main effects are included in a model, but will change if an interaction effect is included, if this interaction effect is nonzero.

Some researchers deal with this problem by simply omitting interactions. Then their results do not depend on how the risk factors are coded, but they may misrepresent what's going on.

For that reason, we need to be specific on how the risk factors are coded. Notice that we appended a subscript "C" to each of the risk factors in the equation above. That is, instead of using the raw data, we subtract a reference value from the raw value first, a process called "centering." For the Bayley indices, we chose to subtract 100, because 100 represents a typical performance on these tests. In other cases we could choose the mean or median of the population. For binary data, we code one response as +0.5, and the other as –0.5 so that the reference value is halfway between. When that is done, the estimated equation is as follows (note that we used S-Plus version 6.1 for Windows to estimate the equations, but any standard statistical package including the capabilities will suffice):

$$\begin{aligned}\text{LO(Low IQ)} = 0.591 - 0.0565^{*}\cdot\text{MDI12}_C - 0.0104\cdot\text{PDI12}_C \\ + .0058\cdot\text{MDI12}_C\cdot\text{PDI12}_C\end{aligned}$$

Ignoring the intercept, we have added asterisks to the coefficients that are statistically significant at the 0.01 level. Only the coefficient associated with the Bayley Mental Development Index (MDI12_C) is nonzero. [Note: the others have estimated values different than zero, but again, we are only considering them "nonzero" if they are statistically significantly different than zero.] If the Bayley mental and motor development indices were overlapping, we'd see one of two things: either *both* the main effects (B_1 and B_2) would be nonzero, or the interaction effect (B_3) would be nonzero (i.e., both risk factors matter when predicting the outcome simultaneously). Since here we see only one of the main effects being nonzero, the two Bayley indices are *not* overlapping.

Finally, we also need to look at the three highly correlated measures of ethnicity. If we fit a logistic regression equation to each of the three pairs of risk factors, we have the following three equations (note that in these three equations, the coefficient of the interaction could not be estimated because it was too strongly correlated with the main effects):

$$\text{LO(Low IQ)} = -0.150 - 0.261\cdot\text{Black}_C + 2.14^{*}\cdot\text{Minority}_C$$
$$\text{LO(Low IQ)} = -0.192 + 0.261\cdot\text{Hispanic}_C + 1.88^{*}\cdot\text{Minority}_C$$
$$\text{LO(Low IQ)} = 0.922 + 1.88^{*}\cdot\text{Black}_C + 2.14^{*}\cdot\text{Hispanic}_C$$

In the first two equations, we find that the main effect for minority is nonzero when included with either black or Hispanic, but the main effects for black or Hispanic are essentially zero. Thus, minority is not an overlapping risk factor with either black or Hispanic. However, in the third equation, the main effects for both black and Hispanic are nonzero, indicating they are overlapping with each other in their ability to predict the outcome.

When two risk factors are found to be overlapping, the challenge is to identify one risk factor that represents the common construct as well as possible. In some cases, that might mean averaging the two, but in other cases, when the two are measured on different scales, averaging them would make no sense. In some cases, we would choose the best of the two—easiest to measure, most reliable, most sensitive—and set aside the other. In some cases, we might use the logistic weights to construct a new measure. For example, we could use 1.88·Black + 2.14·Hispanic as a new composite score, but such a score is not very meaningful. (What does it mean to be 1.88 times black and 2.14 times Hispanic?) In some cases, the fact that the two are overlapping might inspire the researchers to use a completely different risk factor that might focus more directly on the common construct. In short, the strategy would be to somehow reduce the two overlapping risk factors to one, but how exactly to do that may vary from situation to situation and requires specialized knowledge of the application.

In the case of these IHDP data, combining black and Hispanic has already been done for us. If you recall, the risk factor "minority" was actually a risk factor indicating that the individual either self-reports his or herself as black *or* Hispanic, and combining black and Hispanic as above in essence gives us "minority." Thus, we will use the minority risk factor as the composite of black and Hispanic and set black and Hispanic aside.

Also within Each Time Period, Set Aside Proxy Risk Factors

When an outcome has a strong risk factor, any other factor strongly correlated with that risk factor is likely to be a risk factor, even if it has nothing directly to do with the outcome. Thus, if, as often happens, gender is a fixed marker for a disorder (e.g., heart disease, certain types of cancer, depression, schizophrenia), anything strongly associated with gender (e.g., strength, height, weight, number of pregnancies, typical recreational activities—anything that tends to be different, on average, for men and women) would likely be found a risk factor as well, even when the correlate had nothing whatsoever to do with the outcome. Such risk factors are called "proxies." Returning to our path analogy, as shown in Figure 10.3, a proxy is a side road—it leads to the outcome in a roundabout way but only because it intersects with the main route to the destination. Such risk factors are very unlikely to be causal risk factors and serve only to distract attention from factors that may later be identified as causal risk factors. They should be set aside.

Also depicted in Figure 10.3 is the operational definition of a proxy risk factor. Operationally, one risk factor is proxy to another if the two risk factors are correlated, there is no time precedence (or the proxy follows), and when considered simultaneously, the proxy risk factor does not matter. Thus, in the logistic regression model described above, the coefficient of the proxy and the interaction are both essentially zero. [Note: at the end of this chapter, Table 10.4 lists the zero and nonzero coefficients in the logistic regression for each of the five defined inter-actions.]

At this step in our analysis of the IHDP control data, we are looking for proxy risk factors within the same time period (later we will examine those in different time periods). Since we already eliminated black and Hispanic in step 2, the only candidate proxy risk factors within the same time period are the two Bayley indices at one year. Recall that these two indices are highly correlated. Also, recall that when we consider both these Bayley indices and their interaction in the logistic regression equation, only the coefficient corresponding to one of them (the Bayley Mental Development Index—MDI12) was nonzero:

$$\text{LO(Low IQ)} = 0.591 - 0.0565^{*}\cdot\text{MDI12}_C - 0.0104\cdot\text{PDI12}_C + 0.0058\cdot\text{MDI12}_C\cdot\text{PDI12}_C$$

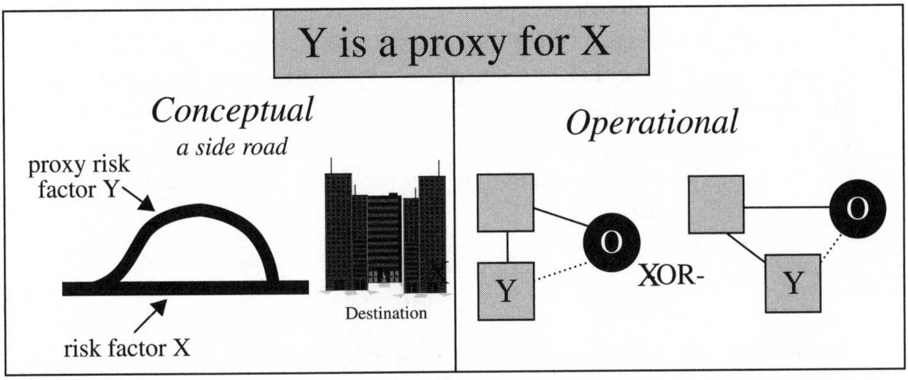

Figure 10.3. An illustration of the conceptual and operational definition of proxy risk factors. The conceptual illustration shows how proxy risk factors are like a side road to a direct road to the destination. The operational illustration depicts X and Y as risk factors and O as the outcome. Left-to-right positioning of X and Y indicates temporal order (here none, or X precedes Y). Solid lines between X, Y, and O indicate correlation, while dotted lines between X, Y, and O indicate correlation that weakens when the other risk factor is considered.

Thus, we will set aside the Bayley Motor Development Index (PDI12) because it is proxy to the Bayley Mental Development Index.

Note that had we chosen to identify proxy risk factors before overlapping risk factors within the same time periods, we would have found that black and Hispanic were proxy to minority and that the Bayley Motor Development Index was proxy to the Bayley Mental Development Index. Only minority at conception and the Bayley mental index at age one would remain, and there would be no more multiple risk factors within the same time period. Then, we would skip identifying overlapping risk factors and be left with the same result as we head into identifying inter-actions *across* time periods.

The Third Step Is to Identify and Set Aside Proxy Risk Factors across Time Periods

Since risk factors can also be proxy to other risk factors that precede them, we now look to risk factors in different time slots to see if there are any additional proxy risk factors. To do so, we check for correlation among pairs of time-ordered risk factors and examine the logistic regression equation that includes both.

Before we check all pairs of risk factors in time order, review in Figure 10.4 the three risk factors that remain: minority, mother's education level at birth, and the Bayley Mental Development Index (in that order). We need to check if mother's education or the mental development index is proxy to minority, or if the mental development index is proxy to mother's education. The first step is to check if these pairs are correlated. From Table 10.2 (and repeated only for these three risk factor in Table 10.3), we find that all three pairs are correlated, and we need to proceed to the next step of estimating the logistic regression equations.

Here are the three estimated regression equations, with the preceding risk factor listed first:

$$\begin{aligned}\text{LO(Low IQ)} = {} & 0.0127 + 1.49^{*}\cdot\text{Minority}_{C} - 0.746^{*}\cdot\text{MomEd}_{C} \\ & + 0.506^{*}\cdot\text{Minority}_{C}\cdot\text{MomEd}_{C}\end{aligned}$$

$$\begin{aligned}\text{LO(Low IQ)} = {} & 0.822 - 0.957^{*}\cdot\text{MomEd}_{C} - 0.0623^{*}\cdot\text{MDI12}_{C} \\ & + 0.00956\cdot\text{MomEd}_{C}\cdot\text{MDI12}_{C}\end{aligned}$$

$$\begin{aligned}\text{LO(Low IQ)} = {} & 0.461 + 2.19^{*}\cdot\text{Minority}_{C} - 0.0598^{*}\cdot\text{MDI12}_{C} \\ & - 0.0245\cdot\text{Minority}_{C}\cdot\text{MDI12}_{C}\end{aligned}$$

In none of these equations is *only* the main effect of the preceding risk factor (the one we list first) nonzero while neither the other main effect nor the

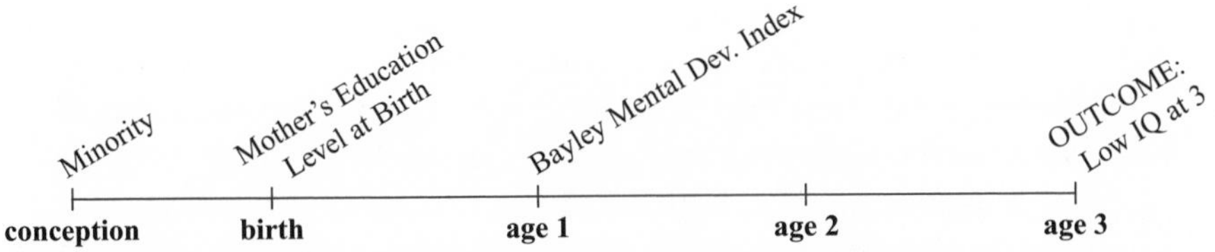

Figure 10.4. The time order of risk factors for low IQ at age three after we remove proxy and overlapping risk factors (IHDP control group).

interaction is nonzero. Thus, there are no proxies among the three remaining risk factors. With these three remaining risk factors, we proceed to the next step: identifying moderators.

The Fourth Step Involves Identifying Moderators and Splitting the Population on the Moderator

One of the most troublesome consequences of the common tendency to omit statistical interactions in, for example, logistic regression equations, is that there is a lack of recognition that the risk factors may be quite different for different subpopulations. For example, the association of age and heart disease is different for men than for women, and the risk factors for sickle cell anemia or Tay-Sachs disease are different for different ethnic groups. When this phenomenon is overlooked and different populations are thrown together ("muddled"), the impact of certain risk factors may be underestimated and the effort to understand how the risk factors might lead to an outcome may be confounded.

Table 10.3
Correlations among the Three Risk Factors for the Outcome Low IQ after We Remove Proxy and Overlapping Risk Factors

	Minority	MDI12
Mother's education	–0.376* ($p < 0.001$)	0.171* ($p < 0.001$)
Minority		–0.170* ($p < 0.001$)

*Statistical significance at the 0.01 level with $r > 0.15$.

Risk factors that moderate the effects of other risk factors identify subpopulations that may have different causal chains leading to the outcome. Recall in the path analogy (see Figure 10.5), a moderator is like a fork in the road; the path to the outcome is different on one fork than on the other.

Operationally, one risk factor moderates another if the two risk factors are *not* correlated, one risk factor precedes the other, and within the subgroups defined by the preceding risk factor, the potency of the other risk factor differs. Although the last part of this operational definition appears to diverge from the definitions of the other operational inter-actions we have described, identifying moderators uses the same logistic regression equation. We can identify a moderator when the correlation and time precedence requirements are met and the interaction effect in the logistic regression equation is nonzero.

Recall from Table 10.3 that all of our three remaining risk factors, minority, mother's education at birth, and the Bayley Mental Development Index, are correlated. Thus, we have no moderators in this example.

Although given our example, we will skip this step, the process of identifying moderators is similar to identifying proxies, except that instead of estimating logistic regression equations with main and interaction effects for all pairs of *correlated* risk factors such that one of the risk factors precedes

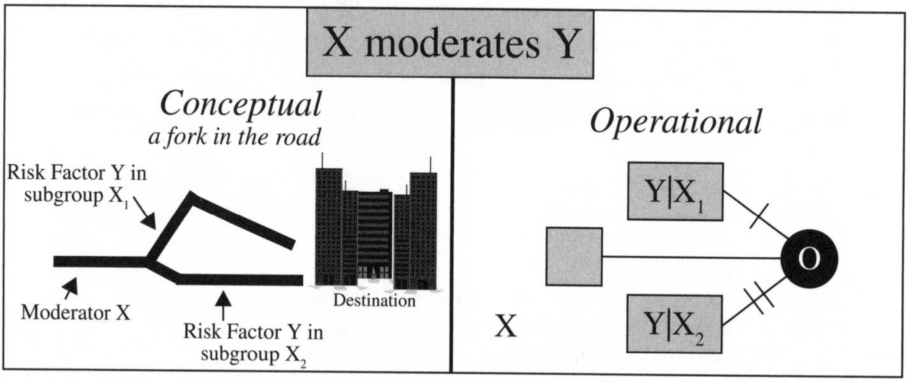

Figure 10.5. An illustration of the conceptual and operational definition of a moderator. The conceptual illustration shows how a moderator is like a fork in the road; the path to the outcome is different on one fork than on the other. The operational illustration depicts X and Y as risk factors and O as the outcome. Left-to-right positioning of X and Y indicates temporal order (here X precedes Y). $Y|X_1$ and $Y|X_2$ indicate the risk factor Y within subgroups of X. The different numbers of slashes on the lines indicate that the relationship between the risk factor Y and the outcome is different within the subgroups of X.

the other, to identify moderators we estimate logistic regression equations for all pairs of *uncorrelated* time-ordered risk factors. If in any of these equations the interaction effect is statistically significantly different than zero, we have identified a moderator.

Once we identify a moderator, we should split the data on the moderator and continue the analysis within each subgroup separately. Thus, if minority had moderated the Bayley Mental Development Index, we would have done the rest of the analysis on minorities and nonminorities separately. In fact, it would probably be a good idea to redo the analysis from scratch within each subgroup since we may discover risk factors in one population that were not previously risk factors in the overall population.

Finally, what if the moderator isn't a simple binary risk factor? For example, suppose we discovered that mother's education (a five point scale) was a moderator of the Bayley Mental Development Index. Then we would stratify the population logically, taking into account sample sizes within each subgroup. For example, if we had enough people, we could do the analysis five times—one time for each of the five mother's education categories. In so doing, we may notice that the results within the lower two and within the upper three look very similar. Then we may combine these and describe two subpopulations based upon the mother's education. If in the new analyses within the two subpopulations we are not seeing mother's education reemerge as a moderator, we have probably split the population appropriately. Unfortunately, this process may take some trial and error as well as some insight into logical ways to stratify the population on the moderator.

The Fifth and Last Step Is to Identify Mediators

Infectious diseases aside, disorders are generally not the result of one and only one causal factor: one gene, one environmental exposure, or one biological entity. And even when they are, there may be multiple paths leading to that one causal factor. For example, AIDS has one cause: the HIV virus. However, there are still many ways an individual is exposed to that causal factor. The different risk factors for AIDS, such as homosexuality, country of origin, and hemophilia, form different chains ultimately leading to the final causal factor and finally to the outcome. Thus, there is typically more than one chain of risk factors, some possibly causal and some not, that leads to a disorder. The links in such a chain are suggested by mediators.

In our path analogy, a mediator is a bridge between a road and the outcome (see Figure 10.6). You must cross the bridge to reach the outcome. In total mediation, the bridge is the only way to get from the risk factor to the outcome (i.e., the mediator totally explains why the mediated risk factor leads to the outcome); in partial mediation, there are other ways the risk factor leads to the outcome (i.e., the mediator explains why the mediated risk factor leads to the outcome, but there are also other explanations).

Operationally, a risk factor mediates another if the two risk factors are correlated, the mediator *follows* what it mediates, and when considered simultaneously, only the mediator matters (total mediation) or both risk factors matter (partial mediation). Again, we return to the logistic regression equation to identify the last requirement. In mediation (total or partial), either the coefficient associated with the mediator *or* the coefficient associated with the interaction is nonzero. Total mediation describes one special case when *only* the coefficient associated with the mediator is nonzero (the other are both zero). Except for this special case, all other cases when the requirements are met for mediation describe partial mediation.

The final step in identifying the inter-actions for the remaining three IHDP risk factors (minority, mother's education, and the Bayley Mental Development Index) is to see if any of these risk factors form mediator chains. If they do not, then they are independent links to low IQ.

We already know the first requirement of correlation is met for all ordered pairs (see Table 10.3). So now all we have to do is check the logistic regression equations we already estimated when we were checking if any risk factors were proxies to risk factors that preceded them. Remember that we

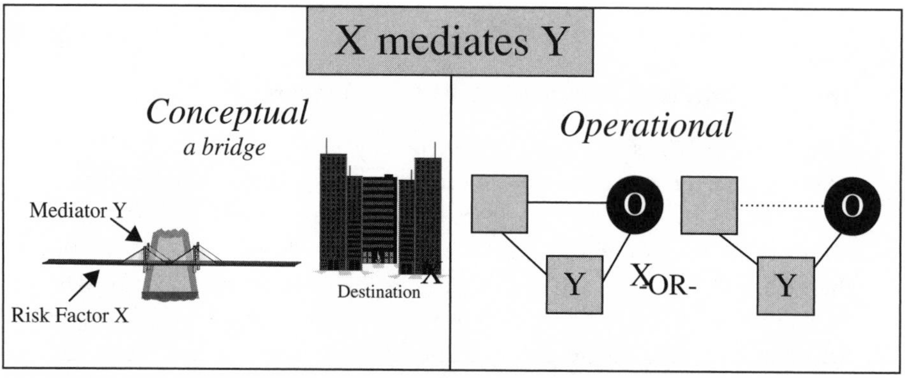

Figure 10.6. An illustration of the conceptual and operational definition of a mediator. The conceptual illustration shows how a mediator is like a bridge between a road and the outcome. The operational illustration depicts X and Y as risk factors and O as the outcome. Left-to-right positioning of X and Y indicates temporal order (here X precedes Y). Solid lines between X, Y, and O indicate correlation, while dotted lines between X, Y, and O indicate correlation that weakens when the other risk factor is considered.

listed these risk factors in time order such that the first risk factor (e.g., minority) precedes the second one listed (e.g., MomEd).

$$\begin{aligned}\text{LO(Low IQ)} = {} & 0.0127 + 1.49^{*}\cdot\text{Minority}_C - 0.746^{*}\cdot\text{MomEd}_C \\ & + 0.506^{*}\cdot\text{Minority}_C\cdot\text{MomEd}_C\end{aligned}$$

$$\begin{aligned}\text{LO(Low IQ)} = {} & 0.822 - 0.957^{*}\cdot\text{MomEd}_C - 0.0623^{*}\cdot\text{MDI12}_C \\ & + 0.00956\cdot\text{MomEd}_C\cdot\text{MDI12}_C\end{aligned}$$

$$\begin{aligned}\text{LO(Low IQ)} = {} & 0.461 + 2.19^{*}\cdot\text{Minority}_C - 0.0598^{*}\cdot\text{MDI12}_C \\ & - 0.0245\cdot\text{Minority}_C\cdot\text{MDI12}_C\end{aligned}$$

Since the coefficient associated with the later risk factor and/or the interaction is nonzero in all three cases, all three of these equations satisfy the third requirement for mediation. Since the coefficient associated with the mediated risk factor (the first one listed) is also nonzero, each of these equations describes a partially mediated risk factor. This chain of three risk factors, depicted in Figure 10.7, suggests that minority status leads (in part) to low education (again, in part) leads to poor mental development of the child, which ultimately culminates in the child's low IQ at three years of age.

Conclusion and Summary

If risk researchers don't follow the model of the prospector who carefully attempts to remove the sand and silt from his sample to produce the "pur-

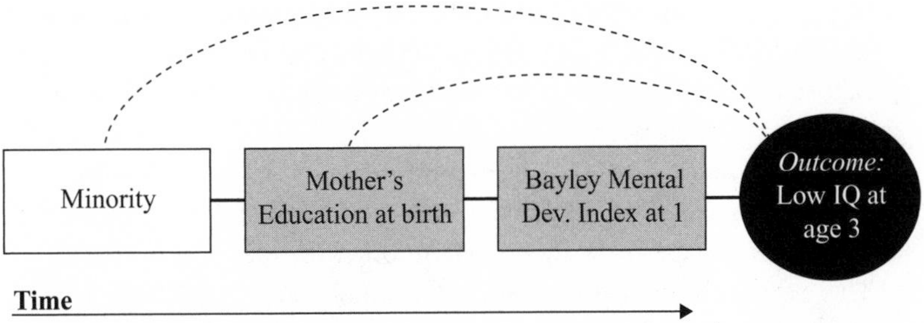

Figure 10.7. The mediator chain leading to the outcome of low IQ at age three among low-birth-weight premature children. The unshaded box is a fixed marker; the shaded boxes are variable risk factors (possibly causal?). The solid connecting lines indicate correlation; the dashed connecting lines indicate correlation that weakens when other factors are considered. The Bayley Mental Development Index mediates the mother's education at birth, which mediates minority. Only minority is a fixed marker; thus, the other two risk factors suggest areas where interventions could be considered.

est" sample of potential gold, then they may become so "weighed down" with all the debris of redundant and inconsequential risk factors that they cannot even isolate any gold from among the muck. The process of examining the relationship among pairs of risk factors, using the concepts and techniques of precedence, correlation, and simultaneous prediction, provides risk researchers a hope of finding what they are really looking for: causal risk factors and causal chains of risk factors that ultimately may illuminate what leads to a disorder and how to prevent it.

At the end of an analysis such as we described, the prospector is ready to bring his find to the assayer to see what the value of his find is. Looking at Figure 10.7, we begin to get some idea of which risk factors are important, how these risk factors fit together, and, specifically looking to the mediator chain, how interventions might be designed to "break the chain" and prevent (or promote) the outcome.

However, one crucial piece of determining the "value" of multiple risk factors remains missing. What we learn from Figure 10.7 motivates future research, but it does not tell us how to identify, on the basis of multiple risk factors, who within the population is at high risk and who is at low risk. Thus, Chapter 11, our final chapter in Part III, describes another methodology to use multiple risk factors to optimally determine high and low risk groups.

- Risk research has a tradition of accumulating risk factors and then counting or scoring them to predict an individual's risk of an outcome. Instead, we recommend identifying the ways risk factors work together to set aside risk factors that are overlapping or proxy to other risk factors in order to find the moderators and mediators.
- Before beginning a moderator–mediator analysis, we need to identify the true risk factors.
- The three main pieces of information necessary for a moderator–mediator analysis are time precedence, correlation, and how a pair of risk factors simultaneously predict an outcome (see Figure 10.8).
- These three components necessary for a moderator–mediator analysis can be obtained (respectively) by time ordering the risk factors, estimating the correlation (ideally Spearman rank correlations) among all pairs of risk factors, and then ascertaining what matters to the outcome by, for example, estimating logistic regression equations with the outcome as the dependent variable and the pair of risk factors (including their statistical interaction) as independent variables.
- First, identify and combine overlapping risk factors and set aside proxy risk factors. (This can be done in either order.) Next see if there

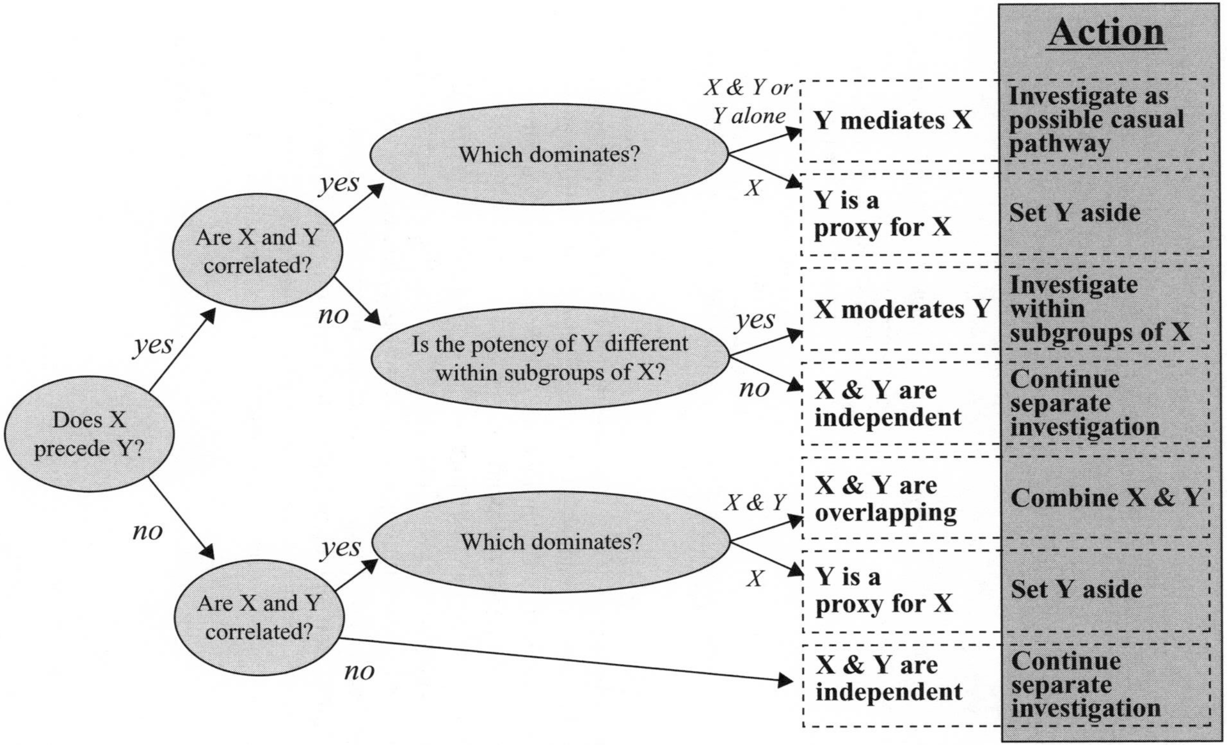

Figure 10.8. A flowchart for determining what inter-action exists between two risk factors, X and Y, for the same outcome. If there is precedence, then define X to be the preceding risk factor. Otherwise, define X to be the dominant risk factor. A risk factor X dominates another risk factor Y if, when used together in simultaneous prediction of the outcome, only X matters. When both risk factors matter in simultaneous prediction, the risk factors "codominate."

Table 10.4
The Requisite Components to Determine Which Inter-action Exists between a Pair of Risk Factors for the Same Outcome

	X and Y Correlated?	X precedes Y?	Logistic Regression Equation: LO(outcome) = $B_O + B_1 \cdot X_C + B_2 \cdot Y_C + B_3 \cdot X_C \cdot Y_C$
Y is proxy to X	Yes	Yes or no	$B_1 \neq 0$ and $B_2 = 0$ and $B_3 = 0$
X and Y overlap	Yes	No	Any two of B_1, B_2, B_3 are $\neq 0$ or B_3 by itself $\neq 0$
X moderates Y	No	Yes	$B_3 \neq 0$
Y mediates X	Yes	Yes	Total: $B_1 = 0$ and $B_3 = 0$ and $B_2 \neq 0$ Partial: any two of B_1, B_2, B_3 are $\neq 0$ or B_3 by itself $\neq 0$
X and Y are independent	No No	No Yes	No requirements $B_3 = 0$

As in Figure 10.8, to use this table, define X as the preceding risk factor. If no risk factor precedes the other, then define X as the dominant risk factor.

are any moderators. If there are, split the data into subpopulations defined by the moderator and start the analysis over within each subpopulation. Finally, identify chains of mediators. Any other risk factors remaining are independent.

- Table 10.4 is a tabular alternative to Figure 10.8 that summarizes the requisite components for identifying each of the five inter-actions for a pair of risk factors if using logistic regression. Here we describe how the risk factors simultaneously predict the outcome (i.e., domination or codomination defined in Figure 10.8) by listing which coefficients of a logistic regression equation are zero or nonzero. The logistic regression equation predicts the outcome using the pair of risk factors.

11

How Do We Use Multiple Risk Factors?

ROC Tree Methods

The legend of St. Denis, the patron saint of Paris, describes how, after St. Denis was martyred by decapitation, he walked two miles carrying his head in his hands. Centuries later, a wise French woman, Mme. Du Deffand (1697–1780), pointed out: "*La distance n'y fait rien, il n'y a que le premier pas qui coute.*" Loosely translated: "The distance doesn't matter—it's only the first step that counts." In short, the miracle is that first step. Once that is taken, all he had to do was repeat it.

In Chapter 9 we described a "first step": establishing the potency of a risk factor by acknowledging *both* the benefit and harm of using a risk factor to predict an outcome. In doing so, we noted that individual risk factors by themselves often are not very potent. Instead, we argued, we must consider multiple risk factors. In Chapter 10 we addressed how multiple risk factors might work together in order to both understand what leads to an outcome and begin to devise ways of preventing (or promoting) it. However, in the end, we had identified which risk factors were important and how they fit together over time but had ignored almost entirely how strong the prediction was.

Now we bring these two issues together by considering potency with respect to multiple risk factors. We describe how to repeat that first step of selecting the most potent risk factor sequentially for multiple risk factors with the ultimate goal of defining groups of high risk and low risk based upon multiple risk factors.

Moderator–mediator analysis allowed us to pare down and organize the list of risk factors as well as gain insight into how the risk factors work together to produce an outcome. However, in addition, the pared down list provides a starting point for the iterative process we describe in this chapter. In this iterative process (called "recursive partitioning"), we select the "best" risk factor to split the population into two groups, and then we select the "best" risk factor within each group, repeating this selection and splitting until a stopping criterion has been met. Each final subgroup consists of individuals at high, low, or moderate risk.

What Is Recursive Partitioning?

The iterative process of splitting the population into two groups, and each group into two more groups, and so forth, can best be graphically represented by an upside-down tree. The top "node" (or "root") depicts the entire sample, representing the entire population. Then the top node "branches" into two nodes, and each such node branches once again into two more nodes, and so on. Figure 11.1 depicts the beginning of one such tree using the Infant Health and Development (IHDP) data[1] we described in Chapters 3, 9, and 10.

The procedure we use to "grow" this tree (often referred to as a "decision tree" or a "classification tree") is one type of recursive partitioning. There are many (at least 30 to our knowledge) such procedures available. The best known and most easily commercially accessible recursive partitioning procedure is called classification and regression tree (CART) analysis.[2] These various procedures differ from each other on (at least) three dimensions:

1. At each node, what criterion determines the next best split?
2. When can a node split no more (the "stopping rule")?
3. What philosophy guides growth and "pruning"—that is, do we attempt to create a very large tree and then possibly trim it back (or "prune it"), or do we attempt to grow only branches that we intend to use, without any pruning?

The version of recursive partitioning we use and recommend (the ROC tree method[3]) is unique in choosing a criterion based on acknowledgment of the relative costs of false positives versus false negatives. We use the weighted kappa coefficient to determine the optimal split at each node. Many of the other recursive partitioning methods do not use a measure of potency to

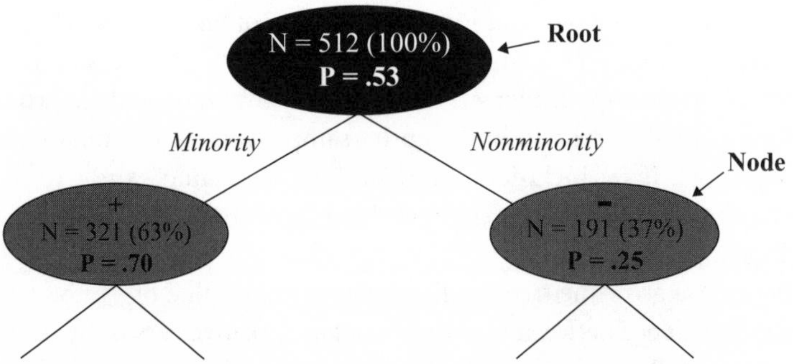

Figure 11.1. The first split for the outcome of low IQ at age three among a sample of low-birth-weight children. For each node, we list the sample size of the subgroup (e.g., $N = 512$), the percentage of the overall population that subgroup represents (e.g., 100%), and the risk in that subgroup (e.g., $P = 0.53$). Each node has a plus (+) or minus (–) to indicate whether it is a higher risk or lower risk node than its parent node.

determine the optimal split; instead, they select the risk factor with the most statistically significant relationship with the outcome.

In the ROC tree method, to split a node further, (1) the node must have a large enough sample size and (2) the risks of the outcome for the two groups created by branching are statistically significantly different from one another. Not satisfying the latter criterion is a typical stopping rule for many of the different methods.

Finally, the ROC tree method tries to grow the most compact tree possible and uses no pruning procedures. A publicly available program to build a decision tree using the ROC tree method can be found at www: toyourhealthbook.com.

How to Grow and Interpret an ROC Tree

In Figure 11.1, we showed the first split of an ROC tree using the risk factors for low IQ at age three from the IHDP data. The risk factors we use are the ones that remain after we have pared down the list of risk factors by combining overlapping risk factors and setting proxy risk factors aside (i.e., minority, mother's education at birth, and the Bayley Mental Development Index at age one). Although we could have used all eight risk factors we started with before paring down the list, we would probably spend unnecessary time and effort dealing with and attempting to interpret splits on proxy or overlapping risk factors. We might miss some important risk factors because we had neglected to combine overlapping risk factors to obtain a more reliable risk factor representing their common construct. Had we identified a moderator, we might attempt growing a tree within each moderated subgroup, or we could grow the tree within the entire sample with moderators included as risk factors. If we include the moderators, we would expect to see the moderator as a branching risk factor and a different branching pattern within the subgroups.

Before we grow the tree, we first must select a value of r to best reflect the relative balance between the harm of a false positive versus the benefit of a true positive. Recall from Chapter 9 that when r is closer to zero, the harm overwhelms the benefit. When r is closer to one, the benefit overwhelms the harm.

First, let's assume the harm and benefits balance out and select $r = 0.5$. Recall from Chapter 9 that the most potent risk factor using Cohen's kappa ($r = 0.5$) for low IQ at age three among the sample of low-birth-weight premature children was "minority" (mother describes child as either black or Hispanic). Hence, if we grow an ROC tree choosing $r = 0.5$, the first branching we see in Figure 11.1 is on minority. Then entire sample ($N = 512$) splits into two nodes: minority ($N = 321$ or 63% of the population) with risk = 0.70 and nonminority ($N = 191$ or 38% of the population) with risk = 0.25. Note that the risk is simply a percentage as well: the percentage of people in that subgroup who will have the outcome (e.g., 70% and 25%). However, to make it easier to separate the percentage of the overall population and the risk, we will write the sample size percentage as a percentage (e.g., 63%) and the risk as a decimal (e.g., $P = 0.70$).

Note how far apart the risks in these two nodes are: 0.70 versus 0.25. Now we repeat the process again within the two new nodes as depicted in Figure 11.2. The criteria we have selected to allow each node to split again are as follows: (1) each of these nodes must have at least 10 individuals with *and* without the outcome and 10 individuals with and without the risk factor, and (2) the optimal branching must show statistical significance at a stringent level ($p < 0.001$).

In the minority node, we find that the optimal branching is based on the criterion Bayley Mental Development Index < 115 versus ≥ 115. This creates two new nodes with risks 0.81 and 0.48 (straddling the risk in the parent node of 0.70). In the nonminority node, the optimal branching is based on a criterion mother attended college or not, with risks 0.45 and 0.09 (again, straddling the risk in the parent node of 0.25).

Once again, we repeat the process in each of the four nodes. Notice that the minority/Bayley Mental Development Index ≥ 115 node splits no further, indicating the stopping criteria has been met in that node (i.e., either there

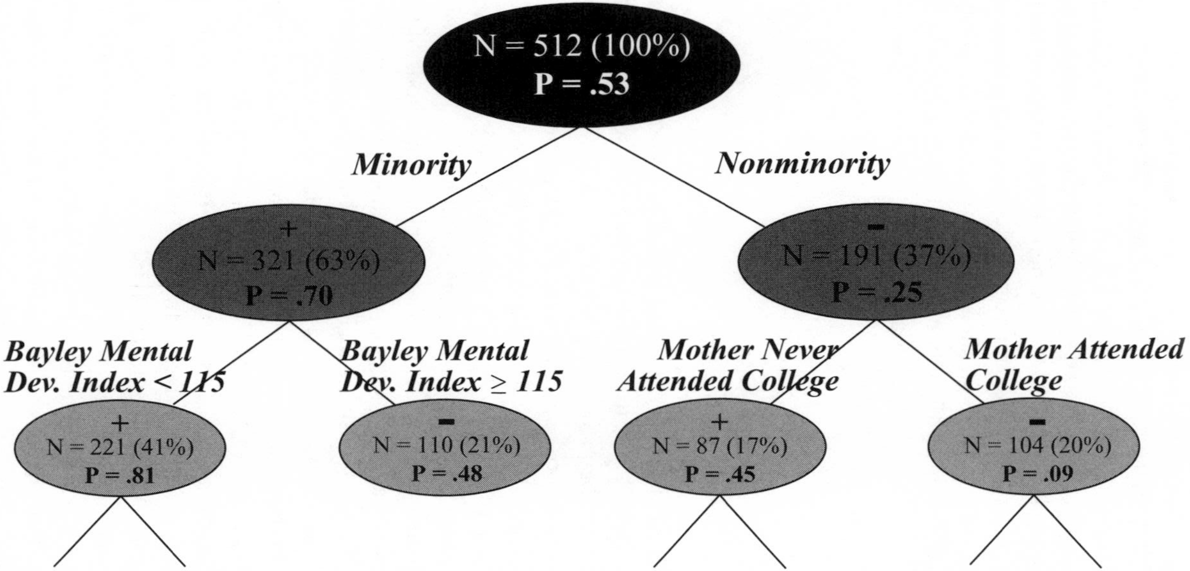

Figure 11.2. The first two splits for the outcome of low IQ at age three among a sample of low-birth-weight children.

are not enough individuals in the node or the optimal split is not statistically significant at the $p < 0.001$ level.). After this third split, the stopping criterion is met in all nodes, and Figure 11.3 depicts the final tree with seven "terminal nodes" or "leaves."

The structure of seven final nodes, with risks of low IQ of (in order) 0.02, 0.19, 0.30, 0.48, 0.65, 0.73, and 0.91, suggests some interesting implications. For example, note that maternal education did not matter in the minority subgroup, but mattered a great deal in the nonminority subgroup. Moreover, the Bayley Mental Development Index mattered both for minorities and low-educated nonminorities, that is, in subgroups disadvantaged in some way, but not in the nondisadvantaged subgroups. These differences might yield strong clues for trying to figure out why each subgroup may be at risk and what might be done to prevent the outcome in each of these subgroups.

Using the ROC Tree to Define the High- and Low-Risk Groups

Now that we have grown the tree and begun interpreting its meaning, we return to the original goal to identify the high-risk subgroup(s) to whom intervention might be provided. To do this, we now assign to each individual in the sample a risk score equal to the risk in the group to which that individual belongs. Thus, all minorities with a Bayley Mental Development Index less than 106 will be assigned a risk score of 0.91, all nonminorities whose mother had graduated from college will be assigned a risk score of 0.02, and so forth. Then, we once again apply the methods of Chapter 9, using the risk score as the risk factor and find the optimal cut point of this new "risk factor" to identify the high-risk individuals when $r = 0.5$. In this case, that cut point is 0.65—that is, the high-risk individuals are those in the three final nodes (leaves) with darker circles around them in Figure 11.3: minorities with a Bayley Mental Development Index less than 115, and nonminorities whose mothers never attended college with a Bayley Mental Development Index less than 106. Those in the high-risk group have risk of low IQ of 0.80, and those in the low-risk group, 0.29. If we chose to deliver intervention to the high-risk group, we would treat 47% of the total population. If the intervention were effective enough to bring the risk of the high-risk group down to the level of the low-risk group, we would reduce the prevalence in the total population from 0.53 to 0.29.

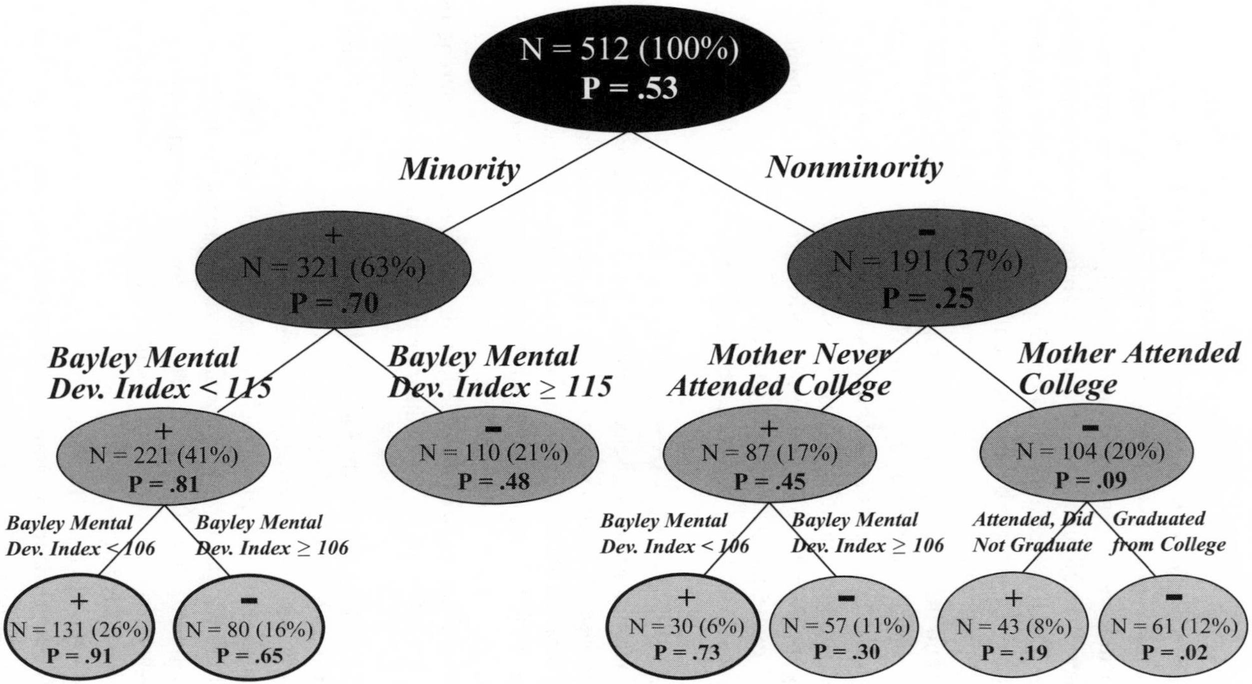

Figure 11.3. The complete ROC tree for the outcome of low IQ at age three among a sample of low-birth-weight children ($r = 0.5$).

Variations in the Harm-to-Benefit Ratio (r) Change the Resulting ROC Tree

Recall that which risk factor is most potent depends on our choice of the harm-to-benefit ratio (r). Recall from Chapter 9 that $r = \$B/(\$B + \$H)$, where \$B and \$H correspond to the costs and risks of correctly identifying someone who will have the outcome and incorrectly identifying someone who will not have the outcome. For example, for an innocuous and inexpensive intervention such as sending early parenting pamphlets home from the hospital with parents of low-birth-weight children, we might choose an r of 0.9—that is, assuming there is some benefit of such an intervention, the cost is low and the potential harm is negligible. On the other hand, the cost of the intervention offered in the IHDP clinical trial was expensive (about \$30,000 per child per year to offer high-quality day care and parental education and support). Although the harm was still probably negligible, the costs of offering the intervention to those who didn't need it were prohibitive. A more appropriate choice of r might be 0.10.

Figures 11.4 and 11.5 depict the resulting trees with $r = 0.1$ and $r = 0.9$, respectively.

As before, using the risk scores described by leaf membership to determine the high-risk group, we select only the group with a risk of 0.95 when $r = 0.1$, and select all groups with a risk of 0.33 or greater when $r = 0.9$. Thus, as summarized in Table 11.1, when we set $r = 0.1$, we would consider 19% of the population to be high risk, while when we set $r = 0.9$, we would consider 80% of the population to be high risk.

The results summarized in Table 11.1, derived from three different trees with $r = 0.1$, $r = 0.5$, and $r = 0.9$, illustrate certain general principles:

- When r is set closer to zero—that is the harm outweighs the benefit—the method leads to setting the risk in the high-risk group as close to one as possible so as to treat only the very high-risk people. The percentage of people in the high-risk group is very low (19% when $r = 0.1$), but their risk tends to be well above the prevalence in the overall population (0.95 vs. 0.53). The risk in the low-risk group (0.44 vs. 0.53 when $r = 0.1$) may be only slightly below the prevalence in the overall population.
- When r is set to 0.5—that is, the harm and benefit are about equal—the method leads to spreading the risk in the high-risk groups and the low-risk groups as far apart as possible. The percentage of people in the high-risk group (47%) usually approximates the prevalence (53%) in the overall population. The risk in the high-risk group and the risk

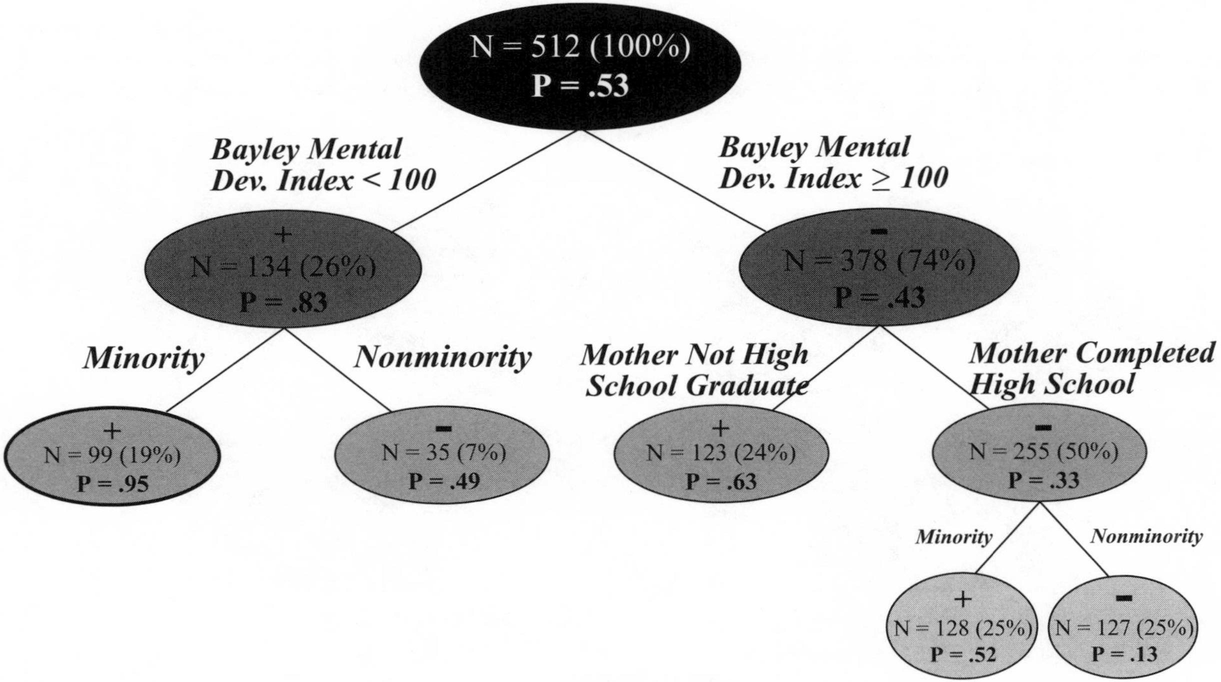

Figure 11.4. The ROC tree for the outcome of low IQ at age three among a sample of low-birth-weight children (r = 0.1). The choice of r closer to zero reflects the high costs of providing the intervention to those identified as high risk (i.e., we want to minimize false positives).

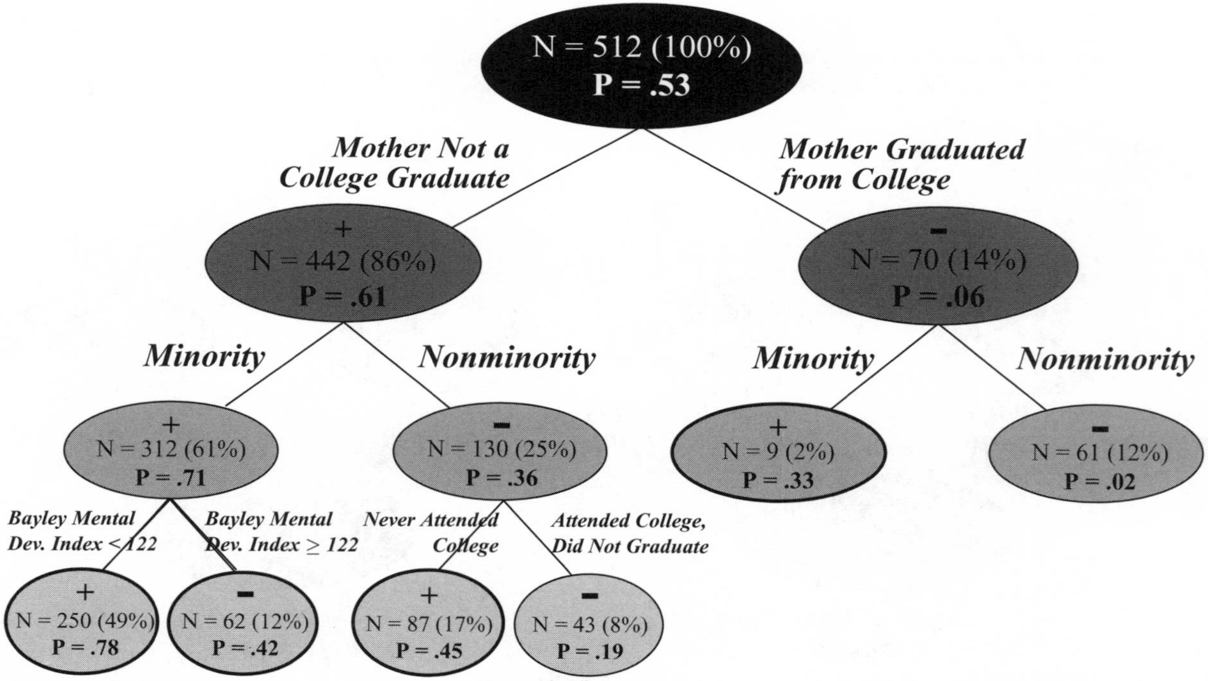

Figure 11.5. The ROC tree for the outcome of low IQ at age three among a sample of low-birth-weight children ($r =$ 0.9). The choice of r closer to one ignores the high costs of providing the intervention to those identified as high risk and instead acknowledges that the benefit is great and the actual harm is negligible.

Table 11.1
The Proportion Considered High and Low Risk and the Risk in the High- and Low-Risk Groups Using Three Different ROC Trees

	High-Risk Group		Low-Risk Group	
	%	Risk	%	Risk
All low risk	0%	N/A	100%	.53
$r = 0.1$	19%	.95	81%	.44
$r = 0.5$	47%	.80	53%	.29
$r = 0.9$	80%	.64	20%	.09
All high risk	100%	.53	0%	N/A

in the low-risk group are spread as far apart as possible—0.80 versus 0.29—straddling the prevalence of 0.53.

- When r is set closer to one—that is, when benefit far outweighs harm—the method leads to obtaining a risk in the low-risk group as close to zero as possible. If we were to treat those in the high-risk group, everyone would be treated except the very low-risk people. Then the percentage of people in the high-risk group is very high (80% when $r = 0.9$), but their risk (0.64) tends to be only slightly above the overall prevalence (again, 0.53) while the risk in the low-risk group (0.09) is usually well below the prevalence. Using an ROC tree with an r close to one is sometimes called a "rule out" decision rule—the only people not recommended for treatment are those at very low risk.

Obviously, it makes a great difference to the number of individuals who would receive treatment, to the level of risk in that group, to the cost of any program devised to deliver that treatment, and ultimately to how much difference that would make to the overall population risk, what value of r is selected to represent the harm-to-benefit ratio.

How Is Growing an ROC Tree Different Than the More Standard Ways of Predicting Outcomes with Multiple Risk Factors?

What we have presented here is, in many cases, a novel way of splitting a population into a high-risk and low-risk group. Currently, the more "standard" way of looking at multiple risk factors is with logistic regression analysis (LRA) or multiple discriminant analysis (which yields similar results to LRA).[4,5] Here we discuss how using LRA compares to growing an ROC tree.

We discussed the basic idea of LRA for pairs of risk factors in Chapter 10. There the log odds of the outcome is a linear model of the two risk factors and their interaction. Could we not extend that idea to deal with, not merely two, but many risk factors simultaneously?

With two risk factors, we estimated four coefficients: the intercept, the two main effects, and the two-factor interaction effect. With three risk factors we would need to estimate eight coefficients: an intercept, three main effects, three two-factor interactions, and a three-factor interaction ($2^3 = 8$). With four risk factors, we would need to estimate 16 ($2^4 = 16$), and so on. Thus, if we had skipped the step where we pared down the number of potential risk factors by identifying "inter-actions" (see Chapter 10) and started to use this approach with the original eight risk factors, we would have had to estimate $2^8 = 256$ coefficients! To estimate that number of parameters requires a very large sample size, perhaps 10 times as many study participants as parameters, here 2,560. The IHDP, which used multiple sites to generate a large sample size, had fewer than half that number.

Accordingly, users of LRA do not usually estimate so many coefficients. Instead, they typically they set most, and frequently all, the interaction coefficients equal to zero and estimate only the remaining coefficients. Thus, for two risk factors they would estimate and interpret three coefficients, for three risk factors they would estimate four, and for the eight risk factors they would estimate nine coefficients—a much less daunting task than estimating 256.

However, interaction effects are often the most important source of information. To omit them from consideration often means the results are incomplete and possibly misleading. When researchers grow ROC trees, they often see evidence of two-way, three-way, and higher way interactions. The influence of maternal educational level on the risk differs between minority and nonminority children, and that the role played by the Bayley Mental Development Index differs depending both on ethnicity and maternal education are missed when interaction effects are not included.

In the end, both the LRA and the ROC tree methods produce a risk score for each individual estimating the risk of that individual having the outcome. In LRA, that risk score is determined by applying the estimated parameters to the observed risk factor values for each individual. In the ROC approach, that risk score is determined by the estimated risk of the leaf matching that individual's profile of risk factors. In both cases, an optimal cut point of risk scores can be computed such that individuals with a risk score exceeding the cut point are classified as high risk.

However, LRA includes no consideration of the possibly different costs of true and false positives (i.e., benefits and harms), in effect, always assuming that harms and benefits balance. The results of LRA often best correspond to those obtained in ROC trees when r is set at 0.5.

In the LRA approach, however, more may be lost. For example, when we set $r = 0.1$, we found that nonminorities with a Bayley Mental Development Index less than 100 had a risk of low IQ of 0.49, very similar to the 0.52 risk of minorities whose mothers completed high school with a Bayley Mental Development Index greater or equal to 100. Yet if we were to offer interventions to both these groups, the types of interventions that might be effective would probably be very different, despite the similarities of their overall risk. In LRA, if the model fit reasonably well, individuals in these two groups would have very similar risk scores, and there would be no indication that the paths to those risk scores might be very different.[6] No stimulus is then provided to consider the possibility that "one size" of intervention might not "fit all." Indeed, this may be one reason that prevention interventions have in the past had notably weak effects.

However, this isn't to say that LRA is not a valuable tool. On the contrary, LRA can be used (and we recommend its use) for testing any a priori hypotheses of random association between a risk factor, or collection of risk factors and their interactions, and an outcome. ROC methods do not provide such statistical tests. However, what we are saying is that the use of logistic regression for trying to "figure out" what's going on in the data—that is, to generate new hypotheses about relationships among many risk factors, and so on—often misses some of the richness in the data that methods such as the ROC tree method can illuminate. Thus, the LRA should play a very important role in testing the hypotheses generated in the ROC tree method, but is not the wisest choice to replace the ROC tree method in generating hypotheses.

Thus, to test a specific hypothesis generated by ROC tree, the next step would be to take that hypothesis (i.e., which subjects are in the high-risk group) and test it in a new sample from the population, estimating the potency of the now multivariate risk factor. Generally, we would expect to see some "shrinkage"—that is, the potency measure in the validation study is not likely to be as strong as that in the hypothesis-generating study.

Conclusion and Summary

Traditional ways of attempting to see patterns in many risk factors often fail to pick up the intricate interplay of multiple risk factors in producing an outcome. Doing a moderator–mediator analysis was the first step in attempting to understand how these risk factors might work together. However, understanding these relationships among risk factors does not suggest a method for determining who in the population is high risk and best suited for an intervention. We recommend the ROC tree method—a recursive partitioning method based on use of the weighted kappa that takes into account the relative importance of the harm to false positives versus the benefit to true positives. The advantage of the ROC tree method is that through a careful selection of the harm-to-benefit balance (*r*), the high-risk group can be selected to reflect the optimal balance of harm to false positives and benefit to true positives.

- Doing a moderator–mediator analysis to pare down an initial list of risk factors to a short list of nonredundant risk factors is the first step for understanding how multiple risk factors work together to produce an outcome. This process does not, however, tell us how specifically to identify the high-risk group or indicate the clinical significance of the identification.
- We could identify a high-risk group by using an appropriate potency measure [we recommend the weighted kappa coefficient with an appropriate choice of the harm-to-benefit balance (*r*)] and selecting the most potent risk factor and the most potent split of that risk factor into high- and low-risk groups. However, to focus on only one risk factor from the initial list of risk factors ignores important information contained in the others.
- By sequentially selecting the most potent risk factor, splitting the population into two groups, and then selecting the most potent risk factor within the subgroups, we can define a "classification" or "decision" tree that creates subgroups of high and low risk based upon multiple risk factors.
- This sequential process of selecting the most potent risk factor, splitting the population, and then repeating this step until some stopping criterion has been met is called "recursive partitioning." There are many such methods that differ in how they choose the most potent risk factor (often not actually using a measure of potency), what the stopping criteria is, and whether they attempt to grow a "lush" tree and "prune" it back or attempt to grow a compact tree.
- The method we recommend, the ROC tree method, uses the weighted kappa coefficient to select the most potent risk factor to split upon. A stopping criterion is activated when the sample size gets too small or

when there are no further statistically significant splits. This method attempts to grow a compact tree and uses no pruning methods.

- Once a tree is grown, a "risk score" can be assigned to each individual based upon the estimated risk of the node to which that individual belongs. Then, the best cut point for the risk score can be chosen using the same ROC methods.
- How the tree is generated depends upon the choice of the harm-to-benefit ratio (*r*). An *r* closer to zero (when harm outweighs benefit) produces a very small high-risk group with a very high risk—such that only the individuals at highest risk are subjected to the intervention. An *r* closer to one (when benefit outweighs harm) produces a large high-risk group with a risk close to the prevalence in the overall population, such that only the individuals with very low risk are excluded from the intervention. An *r* in the middle (0.5) tends spread the risk apart such that the low- and high-risk groups are well differentiated with respect to their risk, and typically the number considered high risk matches the prevalence in the overall population.
- The ROC tree method (as well as all recursive partitioning methods) is a hypothesis-generating method: additional studies are required to test the hypotheses it generates. How well it estimates risk can be tested in a study with a new sample (although shrinkage in the potency is to be expected).

IV

Where Do We Go from Here?

As we said at the beginning of this book, Part IV is our own call to action. We start by stepping back in Chapter 12 to examine and summarize all previous chapters, to remind readers of the main points of those chapters and provide one "bookmark" location for future reference.

In Chapter 13 on making the best of good studies, we take an optimistic view of current research and how, if organized and presented correctly, this research fits into a larger framework of discovering the causes and ways to prevent diseases and disorders. We then speculate with you in Chapter 14, titled "Hope for the Future," on what we all can do to change the face of future risk research.

12

Where Are We Now?

We concluded the introductory chapter with the following:

> Our overall goal for this book is to make every reader a smart skeptic and thereby encourage a shift in the course of future risk research. Poor-quality risk estimation will persist until all of us understand the process better and until we make it clear that we are no longer willing to see taxpayer or philanthropic money spent on unnecessary or flawed research. We also hope that the ideas and approaches described in this book will reduce the amount of erroneous advice based on unsubstantiated claims and prevent decision makers from enacting policy or individuals taking drastic action without careful consideration of the adequacy of research methods and interpretation. The consequences of poor risk research cannot be ignored when the ultimate cost may be the shortened duration and diminished quality of human life.

We hope that Chapters 1–11 took a step in the right direction toward reaching this goal. Before we turn our attention to where risk research is going and should be going, this chapter steps back and reviews the highlights of what we have presented so far. We do this for two reasons. First, we acknowledge that not all readers have read completely all the chapters up to this point. This summary should provide the gist of what may have been missed to enable everyone to read and understand the final two chapters. Second, even for readers who have read every word, we want to present one "bookmark location" for quick reference. In the glossary we have compiled all the definitions presented in this book. In this chapter we review the most important figures and present two integrated lists of questions to ask when considering a research result.

Clear and Correct Communication Is Vital to Correctly Interpreting and Understanding the Results of Risk Research

Throughout this book we attempt to provide clear and precise definitions of the terms commonly used in risk estimation. The glossary at the back of this book presents the terms we have formally defined.[1] The first time we mention each term here in this chapter, we will italicize it to indicate that its definition is included in the glossary.

We began with the most basic of terms of risk research: *risk, risk factor, causal risk factor,* and so on. Figure 12.1 illustrates these terms and is a figure central to this book.

Making sure a risk factor is really a risk factor (and not a just a *correlate*) and then understanding what type of risk factor it is (*fixed marker, variable marker,* or *causal risk factor*) are requisite to knowing what to can be done with it. Fixed markers and variable markers cannot be sources for interventions—if we can't change the risk factor or if changing the risk factor doesn't change the outcome, then attempting to change the risk factor is futile if our goal is prevention of disease or promotion of health. However, fixed and variable markers are valuable for pointing us in the direction of the risk factors that do matter most: causal risk factors.

How Do We Know When a Risk Factor Matters?

Causal risk factors matter most, but our discussions of clinical significance (Chapters 4 and 9) introduce the concern that, whether causal or not, a risk factor may still not matter much. By our definition, a factor is qualified to be called a correlate when researchers demonstrate a *statistically significant relationship* between a factor and an outcome, and even qualified to be called a risk factor when researchers show that the factor precedes the outcome.

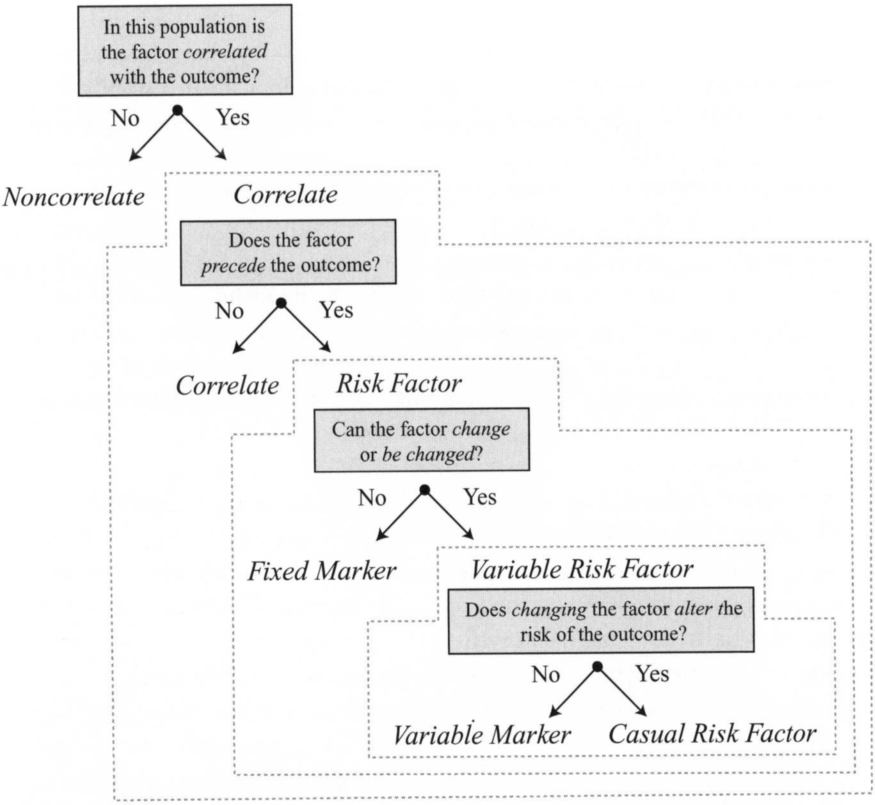

Figure 12.1. Sequential questions to ask to determine whether a characteristic, behavior, environment, or event (a "factor") is a correlate of a specific type of risk factor.

However, even a bona fide risk factor may not be *clinically* significant. If changing a causal risk factor alters the risk of an outcome slightly, but in so doing other problems arise that may outweigh any benefit gained by changing the risk factor in the first place, then more harm than good may result. When risk factors are reported without an accompanying indication of how much they matter (their potency), then just reporting them may likewise do more harm than good.[2]

Unfortunately, measuring and communicating potency is not so simple. Currently, there are many measures of potency, and while some are standard in certain fields, they are not standard across different fields of research and certainly are not easily interpretable by those who are not medical or research professionals. When we are trying to understand the potency of a risk factor, we need to consider the benefit of correctly identifying people who will have the outcome, as well as the harm of incorrectly identifying people who will not have the outcome. *Sensitivity* describes the probability that someone will be correctly identified as high risk (i.e., the probability that someone will benefit from the risk factor), while *specificity* describes the probability that someone will be correctly identified as low risk (i.e., one minus the probability that someone will be harmed). Many of the existing measures of potency, however, trade off this benefit and harm (i.e., sensitivity and specificity) implicitly, and often even the professional presenting the potency measure is unaware of what that implied tradeoff is.

In Chapter 9, we presented a method for visually evaluating potency and comparing different potency measures (receiver operating characteristic, or ROC).[3] In this graphical method, we plot the sensitivity of a risk factor against one minus the specificity. Using these plots, we compared different measures of potency, showing, for example, that even the most commonly used potency measure in risk research (the odds ratio), in some cases, can indicate a very potent risk factor that, in fact, is barely better than random decision making. In addition, we argued that the most informative (and least misleading) potency measure would include consideration of the numbers of people potentially benefited and harmed by being considered high risk, as well as the potential benefit and harm incurred by those people. Since the weighted kappa coefficient is one of the few measures that include both these considerations, we recommend it as the best potency measure for scientific applications. However, for communication with a general audience, we also presented a simple, although less than ideal, way that everyone might begin to comprehend the potency of a risk factor: *number needed to treat/take (NNT)*. The advantage of the NNT is that it fosters consideration of the harm-to-benefit ratio that can be undertaken by anyone to begin to understand whether a risk factor really matters to them.

How Do Risk Factors Work Together?

For many diseases or disorders, researchers have already identified numerous risk factors. For some of these risk factors, researchers have established or could establish their clinical significance—that is, for some purpose, they matter. But even so, armed with this knowledge of many risk factors, some even potent risk factors, why are we are still unable to prevent the outcomes they are associated with?

Although there are probably justified reasons we cannot prevent some diseases or disorders, one aspect of the problem is that, while we know of many risk factors, we do not always understand how these risk factors interrelate and work together to produce the outcome. In Chapter 5 we introduced five terms describing the relationships among two risk factors (*proxy, overlapping, moderator, mediator,* and *independent*).[4] In Chapter 10 we discussed analysis techniques for identifying these relationships. We refer to these types of relationships as "inter-actions" and include a hyphen to differentiate this term from the statistical term "interaction." These relationships are summarized in Figure 12.2.

Extending this pairwise process of identifying the inter-actions to a list of more than two risk factors allows us to pare down a list of risk factors to a core set of few. Most important among this core set are the moderators and mediators. The moderators are instrumental for defining the groups where the results may be different. When these groups are not separated, the results are often blurred. On the other hand, chains of mediators suggest possible causal pathways to be further studied as to whether changing the risk factors in the mediator chains possibly prevents or promotes the outcome. Hence, we call this paring down process "moderator–mediator" analysis, because what we're really seeking are moderators and mediators. A moderator–mediator analysis proceeds as follows:

1. Sort the multiple risk factors by time.
2. For all the risk factors in each time slot, identify and combine overlapping risk factors and set aside proxy risk factors. This leaves only independent risk factors within a time slot. [Note: Usually within each time slot, it does not matter if proxy risk factors or overlapping risk factors are identified first.]
3. For all the now remaining risk factors, examine the relationships between earlier risk factors and later ones. If further proxies are found, set these aside.
4. If a moderator is found, split the population on the moderator and begin the analysis anew within each subgroup defined by the moderator.
5. Finally, for all the now remaining risk factors and possibly within moderator subgroups, examine the relationships between earlier risk factors and later ones to identify mediators.

In Chapter 11 we described how researchers do a moderator–mediator analysis by estimating correlation, determining time precedence, determining how two risk factors *simultaneously* predict an outcome (often using logistic regression analysis). Table 12.1 summarizes the required components for identifying each inter-action.

Once the set of risk factors is pared down to a small set of nonredundant, organized risk factors, the final step for researchers is to use this short list to determine who should be considered at high risk and who should be considered at low risk, and who may be somewhere between. While Chapter 9

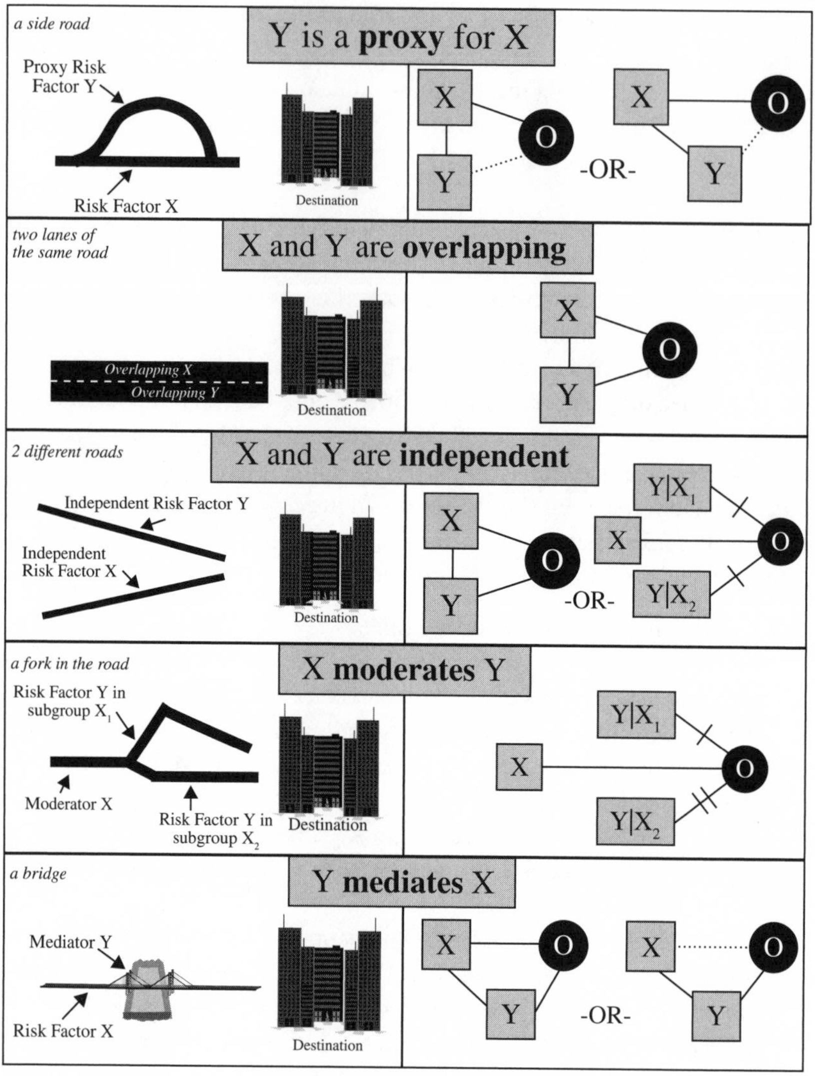

Figure 12.2. An illustration of the conceptual and operational definitions of the five inter-actions. Each of the conceptual illustrations depicts how each of the inter-actions operates along a "route" to the "destination"—the outcome. In each of the operational illustrations X and Y are risk factors; O is the outcome. Left-to-right positioning indicates temporal order. A solid line indicates correlation; a dotted line indicates correlation that weakens when the other risk factor is considered. $Y|X_1$ or $Y|X_2$ indicates the risk factor Y within subgroups of X. The matching slashes on the solid lines indicate that the relationship between the risk factor Y and the outcome is the same within the subgroups of X, unmatching slashes indicate the relationship is different.

Table 12.1
The Requisite Components to Determine Which Inter-action Exists between a Pair of Risk Factors for the Same Outcome

	X and Y Correlated?	X precedes Y?	Logistic Regression Equation: LO(outcome) = $B_o + B_1 \cdot X_c + B_2 \cdot Y_c + B_3 \cdot X_C \cdot Y_C$
Y is proxy to X	Yes	Yes or no	$B_1 \neq 0$ and $B_2 = 0$ and $B_3 = 0$
X and Y overlap	Yes	No	Any two of B_1, B_2, B_3 are $\neq 0$ or B_3 by itself $\neq 0$
X moderates Y	No	Yes	$B_3 \neq 0$
Y mediates X	Yes	Yes	Total: $B_1 = 0$ and $B_3 = 0$ and $B_2 \neq 0$ Partial: any two of B_1, B_2, B_3 are $\neq 0$ or B_3 by itself $\neq 0$
X and Y are independent	No No	No Yes	No requirements $B_3 = 0$

As in Figure 10.8, to use this table, define X as the preceding risk factor. If no risk factor precedes the other, then define X as the dominant risk factor.

focused on determining the "most potent" single risk factor, Chapter 11 focused on how to integrate several risk factors to determine low- and high-risk groups. The method we presented, called the ROC tree method,[3] is one of many "recursive partitioning" methods that takes a population, splits it into two groups using the "best" risk factor, and then splits each of those two groups into two more groups using the most potent risk factor among the subgroups, and so on. The main distinctions between the ROC tree method (publicly available at the Web site www.toyourhealthbook.com) and other recursive partitioning methods (e.g., classification and regression tree analysis[5]) are how the method selects the best risk factor to next split on and when it stops splitting the subpopulations into more subpopulations. The ROC tree method selects the next best risk factor to split on by the weighted kappa coefficient, meaning it includes considerations of the harm-to-benefit ratio. A completed ROC tree run produces subpopulations with distinct risk profiles based on multiple risk factors, allowing anyone to comprehend how having some risk factors and not others might affect an individual's risk of an outcome.

How to Recognize Good and Bad Research

The task of clearly identifying, classifying, and actually using risk factors to predict an outcome should not actually proceed unless the data come from a well-designed research study. Otherwise, the results may be, at best, uninterpretable and, at worst, misleading. Part II of this book is devoted to design and implementation issues, specifically, sampling, design, and measurement.

Throughout this book we have stressed that the population studied is the population to whom the finding should be applied. The crucial question to ask when reviewing a research result is how much like, for example, yourself, your patients, or your constituency, are the participants sampled for that risk study. If the answer is "not very," then the results of that study, no matter how well done, should not be considered for yourself, your patients, your constituency, or whomever you intend to apply the findings to.

However, even when the population studied appears appropriate, how researchers selected the participants is critical to the credibility of the result. We introduced ways of drawing a sample that are likely to produce a valid result: *random sampling, representative sampling, naturalistic sampling,* and *two-stage prospective sampling.* These sampling methods can also be employed at each site of a multisite study, which, if analyzed correctly, may be able to overcome the concerns of population differences across different geographies.

On the flip side, we presented other very common ways of drawing a sample that may very possibly lead to misleading or false results. These ways include all forms of retrospective sampling (including *case-control sampling*) and sampling time instead of people (i.e., the use of incidence rates). Retrospective sampling has three main problems that may lead to an invalid result:

1. The population is likely to be different when researchers start at the outcome and look back than when they start at a time before the outcome has occurred and look forward.
2. Retrospective recall is often unreliable and may even be affected by whether or not the outcome occurs.
3. Researchers may not be able to tell whether the potential risk factor precedes the outcome.

Case-control sampling shares these problems of retrospective sampling, plus, since never in the process of drawing a case-control sample do researchers draw a representative sample, the likelihood that either the cases or the controls are representative of all the cases or noncases in the same population is very low. As we have mentioned many times, generalizing to a population different than the one from which the sample is drawn can be, and often is, very misleading.

We are not saying that case-control studies are not valuable—what is more logical than comparing a group with a disease to a group without and try to figure out differences? What we are saying, however, is that we cannot estimate risk in this way primarily because we are not looking at a population that in any way resembles a representative population—and at the same time, we cannot determine risk factors but can only identify potential risk factors that need to be confirmed in a differently designed study.

In Chapter 6 on sampling, we discussed the problems of defining an outcome in terms of occurrences per time (e.g., person-years) rather than simply occurrences. In this method (which we referred to as sampling people-time), researchers compare the number of "disease-free" years (or days or minutes, etc.) between a treatment and a control group and report an "incidence rate"—the number of events per person-time. Not only is interpreting the results of such a study difficult (what does it mean to say ratio of events per people-year between a control and treatment group is 0.5?), but the rationale for counting multiple years from the same subject as separate entities and pooling these years across subjects stems from a mathematical model called the "constant hazards model." The assumption behind the constant hazard model is simply that the "hazard" is constant, meaning, for example, that if you do not have a heart attack by age 50, your risk of a heart attack in the next year is the same as it was the previous year and is the same as it was when you were age 10, 20, and 30. It's hard to come up with a medical example where the risk does not change with age. Strange results may stem from a model whose basic assumptions are not met.

While we urge studies based on sampling people-time not be considered for use in medical decision making, an alternative that we do advocate is the use of survival methods, in which researchers compare the number of disease-free participants in each of the control and treatment groups plotted against time. These methods are well established and are increasingly being used in situations where participants may be followed for different amounts of time and the outcome may occur at any time throughout the duration of the study.

How researchers collect the sample is closely aligned with how they plan to conduct the study. The most crucial element of study design to check is whether the design allows researchers to draw valid conclusions about the time precedence of any possible risk factor and the outcome of interest. Moreover, does the design allow researchers to draw valid conclusions about causality?

Drawing valid conclusions about the time precedence of risk factors simply requires observing that the risk factor precedes the outcome. For factors that people are born with (gender, race, genetics, etc.), we can assume that they precede the outcome, as long as the outcome occurs sometime after birth. A study that looks at participants once and assesses whether or not they have the outcome of interest (i.e., a *cross-sectional study*) is all that is necessary to establish these factors as risk factors. However, for nonfixed factors (e.g., cholesterol level, anxiety, depression, obesity), the only way to know that the factor precedes the outcome is to have observed the study participant prior to the onset of the outcome and then to have observed whether the outcome occurs or not. This requires a study that is longer in duration and involves at least two (and probably more) evaluations (i.e., a *longitudinal study*). The risk factors of most interest, particularly causal risk factors, are not fixed factors. Thus, to study these factors and establish them as risk factors, longitudinal studies are necessary.

Although longitudinal studies are usually the most valuable types of studies with respect to the information they can provide, they often still cannot provide convincing evidence that a risk factor is causal. How do we know that changing a risk factor alters the outcome when researchers simply observed whether or not an individual has a risk factor and then subsequently has an outcome? The only way researchers can know is by manipulating the risk factor—that is, randomly selecting some people who will have the risk factor changed and seeing if this change affects the risk of the outcome. Such a study is called a *randomized clinical trial* (*RCT*)—an expensive, difficult, and sometimes even impossible study to conduct. Nevertheless, RCTs are the only way to establish causality, in a single, or even in a few, studies. The alternative we described as "a convergence of evidence"—the bringing together of many studies all pointing to the same result and all having a different design such that the source of criticism in one study does not coincide with the source of criticism for another study. The number of studies that constitute a "convergence of evidence" is not clear, but what is clear is that it requires many studies and therefore is both more expensive and more time-consuming than a few well-designed RCTs.

The final question we need to ask ourselves when reviewing a study is whether the risk factors and/or the outcome reported truly reflect what's going on. A diagnosis and a disease, as well as a measurement and a characteristic, are not always the same thing. Just as one of our criticisms of retrospective recall is that the recall may not be what really happened, a measurement of characteristic or a diagnosis of a disease may also be more influenced by who is taking the measurement or making the diagnosis than what the characteristic or disease state is.

All medical research is based on use of measurements and diagnoses, where the inferences are drawn to characteristics and diagnoses of study participants. When done carefully, that is, with due concern for the *reliability* and *validity* of the measurements and diagnoses, this poses no problem. In risk research, in particular, the outcome of interest is frequently some diagnosis, and the risk factors are always based on measurements. The quality of such diagnoses and measurements has a major impact on the credibility of the results.

Often the reliability and validity of the measurements are not at the forefront of criticism of a result, nor is much attention typically paid to reporting the reliability and validity of the measures used. Our message in Chapter 8 is that measurement quality, too, can have an overwhelming influence on the credibility of the result: it can explain why two studies might disagree or why a result might not be statistically significant. Thus, we also need to pay attention to how factors and outcomes are measured and diagnosed and make sure that they were measured reliably and validly.

Finally, to bring together many of the issues we have summarized in this chapter, we present two heuristics, shown in Tables 12.2 and 12.3. One consists of questions to ask when considering whether a study design is relevant to your needs; the other describes what can and cannot be learned from each of different type of study.

Conclusion and Summary

Our aim in this chapter is to provide the reader with a central location to easily review the concepts presented in this book. Hence, we conclude this chapter with a summary of relevant excerpts from each chapter's conclusion and summary.

- *Chapter 1:* When it comes to comprehending the results of risk estimation, the words used either by the original researcher or by anyone describing the result are critical for guiding how we think about and respond to the result. For this reason, we stress to the researcher, the reporter, and everyone considering a result, the importance of correctly using the terms central to risk research.
- *Chapter 2:* The definition of "risk factor" requires that researchers demonstrate the factor precedes the outcome. When researchers cannot establish precedence—typically because they measured the correlate and outcome simultaneously—there is a "chicken-and-egg" problem of figuring out which is the risk factor and which is the outcome. Even when a correlate is correctly described as such, if other researchers, doctors, and medical consumers interpret the correlate as a risk factor (and particularly if they interpret it as a "cause"), they may consider taking action on the basis of misleading information. As a result, research dollars may be wasted because researchers are looking at the wrong outcome, or health might be jeopardized if individuals take action to change a correlate that ultimately has no effect on preventing the outcome.

Table 12.2
Questions to Ask When Reviewing a Research Study

	Okay to Base Decisions on Result	***Warning***	Do Not Base Decisions on Result
1. Are the results statistically significant?	Yes.		No
2. Did the researchers provide evidence of clinical significance?	Yes, in a format that meets your needs	Yes, but the measure may not reflect how you trade off true versus false positives.	No, either the risk factor is not very potent or researchers did not present a potency measure.
3. What population did researchers study?	The population you care about.	A population similar to the one you care about.	A population different than the one you care about.
4. How did researchers select the sample?	Prospectively with evidence that the sample is representative of the target population.	Prospectively, but how representative it is of the target population is questionable.	Retrospectively (e.g , case-control) and/or with a clear bias toward certain individuals.
5. Did researchers conduct the study at multiple sites?	Yes—results were analyzed by site and then combined using a weighting scheme.	No—keep in mind that the results may differ in different places.	Yes, but the results were "muddled" (i e., pooled and then analyzed).
6. How well are the potential risk factors and outcome measured?	There is evidence of reliability and validity of the measures used.	The measures have questionable reliability and/or validity.	Researchers used retrospective recall and/or events were counted per person-year rather than per person
7. Is the study cross-sectional or longitudinal?	*Longitudinal:* See Table 12.3 for what you can learn from each type of study and what to check for.	*Cross-sectional:* Only fixed factors can be called and considered risk factors, and nothing can be called or considered a "cause."	

Table 12.3
What You Can and Cannot Learn from Study Results

	What You Can Learn from Study Results	What You Cannot Learn from Study Results	Things to Check
1. The study is cross-sectional.	Only fixed factors can be called and considered risk factors.	Variable factors cannot be called and considered risk factors or causes.	
2. The study is longitudinal (experimental or observational).	Researchers can establish the precedence of variable factors and, if so established, can call them risk factors	If the study is observational, any identified risk factors cannot be called or considered causal.	Did the study start early enough to capture most of the cases? Were enough cases observed to draw conclusions (at least 50 or so)? Is the drop-out rate low? Did researchers discuss how they dealt with missing data?
3. The study is experimental [i.e., a randomized clinical trial (RCT)].	Researchers can establish whether a risk factor is causal.		Are the three requirements of an RCT met? Specifically: —Is there a control group? —Were study participants randomized into the treatment or control group? —Were the participants and the research staff "blinded" as to who was in the control group and who was in the treatment group? Most important, did the persons who judged whether or not the outcome occurred know who was in which group?

- *Chapter 3:* All risk factors are not equal. Our purpose of classifying the different types of risk factors is to emphasize that although all risk factors can be used to identify those most in need of an intervention and can be used to motivate further research, many, if not most, risk factors cannot be used to prevent or promote an outcome. When we read of an exciting new risk factor, we all need to consider what type that risk factor is before we consider the implications of the finding. Doing otherwise—in particular, assuming a risk factor is necessarily causal—can waste time and money, and possibly can harm.
- *Chapter 4:* Researchers must always take some step beyond statistical significance to communicate why the finding matters. Communicating clinical significance in a way that is more understandable to everyone is simply another vital step to changing the face of risk research.
- *Chapter 5:* When researchers add yet another risk factor to the pile, often the addition doesn't increase our understanding of what promotes health and prevents disease, particularly when many of those individual risk factors by themselves have very little potency. Our best chance of increasing our understanding and further motivating good research is for researchers to pare down the list to the fundamental core of risk factors, rather than confusing issues by accumulating many different risk factors that ultimately may prove to be the same.
- *Chapter 6:* Many of the sampling methods that we urge not be used as a basis for medical decision making—retrospective sampling, case-control sampling, use of incidence rates—are quite common in risk research primarily because they are easier ways to get an answer quickly. In many cases, these quick answers are exactly what researchers need to design better risk studies for future research. Unfortunately, all too often these quick "answers" hit the press and are interpreted as the true answers before additional research is conducted or even considered—as in the 15 years between the initial hormone replacement therapy (HRT) studies and the Women's Health Initiative study on HRT. The fundamental shift in risk research we are urging is a shift from these easier, but also often misleading, ways of collecting a sample to the ones more likely to produce credible and reproducible results.
- *Chapter 7:* The path of least resistance in risk estimation studies is a cross-sectional study: simple, inexpensive, fast, and easy to publish. However, this path is very limited in its yield of results likely to elucidate the causes, prevention, or cures of medical outcomes. A

harder path is longitudinal studies, which are difficult, costly, and time-consuming but the only path to the most valuable risk estimation results for medical decision making. However, such studies still cannot establish causal risk factors. Finally, the hardest path is a special type of longitudinal study, the randomized clinical trial (RCT), the only path that can provide convincing evidence of causality of a risk factor for an outcome. This type of study is particularly important to decision making, in that it documents what interventions might prevent or promote outcomes. While an RCT is expensive and time-consuming, in the end it may not be more expensive or more time-consuming than the multiple, and different, studies required to provide convincing evidence of causality without an RCT. Worse yet, an RCT is also probably not more expensive and time-consuming (and probably less dangerous) than taking action based on results from other studies that were easy, but possibly wrong.

- *Chapter 8:* Anyone evaluating the result of a risk estimation study needs to carefully examine how the diagnosis is made and how the risk factors are measured, by whom, and under what circumstances. Although typically not a lot of information about validity and reliability is provided in journal articles, researchers should provide some assurance that they measured the risk factors and outcome both reliably and validly.
- *Chapter 9:* We have repeated it many times: statistical significance is simply not enough. When researchers move beyond statistical significance and recognize the need to acknowledge both the possible benefits and the possible harms from using a risk factor, they will be motivated to present a measure of potency that communicates both. Many commonly reported measures, notably the odds ratio, fail to explicitly take into account the benefits and harms of true and false identification. We propose that the measure of potency that best communicates both is the weighted kappa coefficient, with the weight reflecting the relative balance of harm to false positives versus benefit to true positives. However, recognizing the challenges in "throwing away" whichever potency measure researchers are most familiar with, we would suggest they also report P, $\kappa(0)$, and $\kappa(1)$, from which a little effort would yield any other measure of association.
- *Chapter 10:* If risk researchers don't follow the model of the prospector who carefully attempts to remove the sand and silt from his sample to produce the "purest" sample of potential gold, then they may become so "weighed down" with all the debris of redundant and inconsequential risk factors that they cannot even isolate any gold

from among the muck. The process of examining the relationship among pairs of risk factors, using the concepts and techniques of precedence, correlation, and simultaneous prediction, provides risk researchers a hope of finding what they are really looking for: causal risk factors and causal chains of risk factors that ultimately may illuminate what leads to a disorder and how to prevent it.

- *Chapter 11:* Traditional ways of attempting to see patterns in many risk factors often fail to pick up the intricate interplay of multiple risk factors in producing an outcome. Doing a moderator–mediator analysis was the first step in attempting to understand how these risk factors might work together. However, understanding these relationships among risk factors does not suggest a method for determining who in the population is high risk and best suited for an intervention. We recommend the ROC tree method—a recursive partitioning method based on use of the weighted kappa that takes into account the relative importance of the harm to false positives versus the benefit to true positives. The advantage of the ROC tree method is that through a careful selection of the harm-to-benefit balance (r), the high-risk group can be selected to reflect the optimal balance of harm to false positives and benefit to true positives.

13

Making the Best of Good Studies

Virtually all researchers are aware of—or should be aware of—the problems of assuming correlates identified in cross-sectional studies are risk factors, of estimating risk with retrospective sampling and retrospective reports, of drawing conclusions about causality from observational rather than experimental studies, and of focusing on statistical significance rather than assessing clinical significance. In none of these areas have we been anywhere close to the first people to point out serious issues. Even the relatively new developments we present—strict scientific terminology, using harm and benefit to assess clinical significance, methods to compare potency of risk factors, and sequential use of these methods to optimally use multiple risk factors—are all solidly based on earlier scientific work. Our approach differs in bringing all these issues together, in having a very low tolerance for conclusions likely to be erroneous and in trying to formulate a better strategy for future risk research.

What exactly is this strategy? After reading all of our cautions about poor research and/or misleading interpretations, you may conclude that you can always find points on which to criticize almost any research result, and start questioning your own fundamental understanding of risk factors and risk research. Perhaps, you may conclude, this strategy should begin with throwing out all previous results and starting over, doing it all "right." But in fact, a lot of good researchers have done and are doing high-quality medical research. We certainly are not suggesting we throw everything out—rather, we need to realize the limitations of past results, consider past research results in the context of those limitations, and move in a more productive direction from this point on.

In that spirit, we devote this chapter to presenting research that, in our view, has been done right. We focus specifically on how these research results fit into the "bigger picture" of assessing risk and ultimately discovering the causes of diseases and disorders and how to prevent them. Selecting particular studies to present here was perhaps our biggest challenge in writing this book—many studies have been done well—but even well-done studies have at times been overinterpreted, whether by the researchers themselves, by the clinicians, or by the media. Each of these studies has value, but each taken alone cannot definitively explain what's going on—particularly for the most complicated of diseases and disorders we care most about, for example, cancer, heart disease, Alzheimer's disease, and mental disorders. Thus, our focus is on how these studies fit into a framework of discovering the causes of complicated diseases or disorders and what needs to precede and follow these studies to definitively describe the risk factors, and particularly the causal risk factors, of the disease or disorder of interest.

We Propose the Following Framework for Considering How Studies Fit Together

No one research project can hope to definitively and conclusively answer any question. At the very least, findings of any one research study need to be replicated and verified before its results become scientific fact. Each well-done research project pushes the limits of our understanding a step or two further and sets up the next research projects to push those limits even further. Thus, each research project provides a few pieces of a puzzle, and if the process of iterative research goes smoothly forward, the entire picture will eventually emerge. However, when steps are skipped or the findings of even the best-done studies are misrepresented and/or misinterpreted, then some of the puzzle pieces are forced into places where they may not belong. Misplaced pieces often delay overall progress toward understanding the whole picture until someone later identifies which pieces were misplaced.

The strategy we describe here is the recognition of how all these pieces should fit together, resulting from a natural progression of research that leads to the right answer as quickly as possible. We suggest that how the Food and Drug Administration (FDA) classifies studies leading to approval of a drug might serve as a model for this strategy. In phase I of drug trials, researchers test the drug in animal models or on small groups of volunteers to evaluate safety and determine appropriate dosages. In phase II researchers continue to test the drug's safety using large samples of people and begin to explore the efficacy of the drug. In phase III, researchers continue to monitor the safety of the drug while studying larger samples of people in randomized clinical trials that test the efficacy of a drug relative to that of other treatments, including placebo. If this phase successfully documents the drug's efficacy, then the drug may be licensed for marketing and the labeling approved.[1]

Similarly we propose three phases of risk estimation. Phase I consists of cross-sectional and case-control studies. Although such studies cannot establish most risk factors, they do provide valuable insights to further investigate in subsequent studies. Specifically, phase I risk studies provide:

- Identification, rationale, and justification to pursue certain potential risk factors
- Guidance as to which populations might be studied
- Guidance for determining an appropriate sample size
- Information about possible measurement issues of the potential risk factors and outcomes

Notice that all this information is very useful for researchers contemplating future research to design the most cost-effective and relevant study. However, very little of this information is appropriate for anyone hoping to use the results to improve their own health or the health of others.

In phase II of risk estimation, we propose that researchers use longitudinal observational studies to establish potential risk factors suggested in phase I and to best identify individuals at high and low risk. However, from such observational studies, no one can assume that changing a risk factor will change his or her risk of the outcome. That must be left to randomized clinical trials. Nevertheless, phase II longitudinal observational studies add valuable pieces to the puzzle in allowing researchers to:

- Establish risk factors
- Remove proxy and combine overlapping risk factors
- Identify moderators to split the population into subpopulations
- Identify mediator chains—the first place researchers should look for identifying potential causal risk factors to study in a future randomized clinical trial

In phase III researchers would typically use randomized clinical trials to establish which variable risk factors are casual risk factors. In this phase, researchers might use the fixed markers and/or moderators identified in phase

II to determine who should be studied or to decide whether and how to divide the population to get the most informative results.

Notice in Figure 13.1 how the three phases we propose correspond directly to the three levels of the hierarchy of studies we presented in Chapter 7. Each of these levels corresponds to one of the phases of risk estimation.

For risk research, we advocate the recognition of these different phases, the recognition of what phase a particular study fits into, and the realization that if a phase is skipped, pieces of the puzzle may be misplaced. If researchers guess what those missing pieces are, they may be simply wrong. Figure 13.1 illustrates how one phase provides the necessary foundation upon which researchers can build the next phase. Proceeding to a subsequent phase before completing the phases before it can be an expensive gamble. Researchers may hit the jackpot and save valuable time and money, but they may also lose more valuable time and money and have "not statistically significant" results because they were missing valuable pieces of information to best design the study. In addition, harm may be done to the participants with no counterbalancing benefit to future patients. When this happens, researchers are faced with the choice of trying again (and possibly failing again), giving up altogether, or simply stepping back and doing the research that should have been done in the first place.

In what follows, we illustrate well-done studies from each of the three phases we propose here and try to describe what came before, what researchers found, how they reported the results, and what should logically follow.

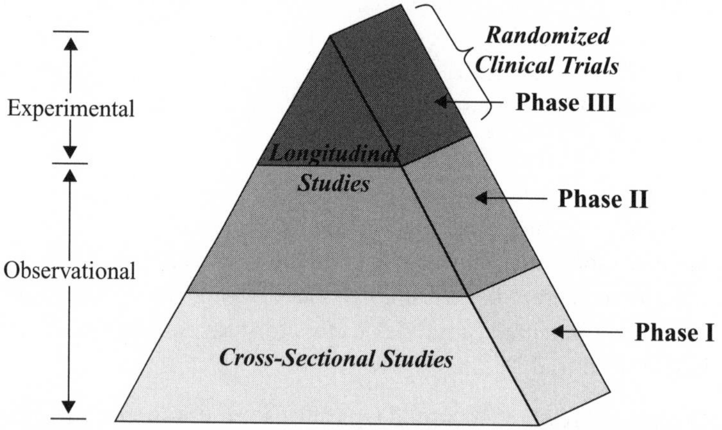

Figure 13.1. How the three phases of risk estimation proposed here correspond to the three levels in the hierarchy of the different types of risk estimation studies.

Phase I: Cross-sectional Studies Are the Foundation of Good Risk Estimation

Cross-sectional studies quickly and easily provide the motivation to pursue certain potential risk factors in a more rigorous (and thus more expensive and time-consuming) study and to dissuade interest in others. Although we have expressed much concern that many people often misuse cross-sectional studies to answer questions beyond their scope, that doesn't in the least discount their value when they are recognized as phase I of risk estimation. Many well-designed cross-sectional studies exist for us to choose from. The problem is often not in the design or analysis but in the presentation, interpretation, and dissemination of the results. Consider Example 13.1, which describes a study that serves as a model in every respect.

EXAMPLE 13.1

Researchers confirmed the hypothesis that "risky" behaviors such as physical fighting, not using birth control, lack of a healthy diet, and use of tobacco were associated with self-reported symptoms of depression.[2] Their study was based on a cross-sectional representative sample of 2,224 9th and 12th grade students in Massachusetts. Thirty-two schools agreed to participate among 50 public schools randomly selected from all high schools in the state. (Comparison of these schools with all public high schools in the state suggested no bias in the selection.) The 2,224 participants were consenting students in one of four classes (two 9th grade, two 12th grade) randomly selected from the mandatory classes offered at each school.

Since this was a cross-sectional study, the researchers could not—and carefully did not—claim that the behaviors studied were risk factors for depression. In fact, to assure that unwary readers did not draw conclusions beyond the scope of what the research demonstrated, they included the following statement in their concluding section:

> The temporal relationship of depressed mood and other risk behaviors cannot be assessed in a cross-sectional data set. The observed associations might suggest that depressed/stressed teens deal with their emotional problems by engaging in risky behaviors. Conversely, teens may find that living a lifestyle that includes multiple risky behaviors leads to feelings of depression/stress. Even in longitudinal data sets, the temporal relationships can be difficult to establish

because emotional problems may have a range of relationships and interactions with adolescent risk behaviors.[1(p245)]

However, this study did establish gender as a fixed marker for depression. As many others have shown, girls are more likely than boys to report stress and depression, particularly at an early age. As seen in this study and others, gender may moderate subsequent risk factors, and the process by which girls become depressed might differ from that of boys. This warns future phase II researchers that they should analyze girls and boys separately.

In addition, this study established age as a variable marker for depression. Of those individuals seen at ages less that 16, a little more than 30% reported depression/stress, rising to about 40% toward the end of the teen years. These ages suggests that longitudinal studies probably should start before or during the early years of puberty to detect the temporal sequence of the implicated behaviors and the onset of depression, and follow these children at least until about age 20.

The researchers point out that the outcome they used was a self-report of depression/stress symptoms, emphasizing that this might differ from a clinical diagnosis of depression, suggesting that researchers conducting a future longitudinal study may want to consider more carefully exactly what outcome is most important and informative and decide carefully how to measure that outcome. Quite appropriately, the researchers end their report with the recommendation for longitudinal studies (phase II studies).

As a measure of potency, they reported a measure we caution against (the odds ratio), as is the convention in this field. The odds ratios they reported were not very strong (in the range of 0.51–1.92). However, these measures of potency were calculated by mixing the varying ages of study participants, and because age was found to also correlate with the outcome, such findings might be different in another study that focused on a particular age or used a more reliable indicator of depression (such as a clinical diagnosis). Nevertheless, since we are not interpreting these correlates as risk factors, having weak indications of potency should only motivate other researchers to do the next phase of the research differently and better.

As described in Example 13.1, what we learn from such well-done cross-sectional studies primarily benefits future research and researchers, not the rest of us who are most interested in how those results matter to us, our patients, our community, and so on. The results may well be intriguing and worthy of consideration, but we all should leave it at that and wait until researchers conduct further phases of the research.

Similarly, those studies that use a case-control sampling scheme are a necessary component of phase I when the outcomes are rare. Otherwise, researchers would have to spend too much money to get a representative sample for a study. However, given the problems inherent in case-control studies, they should never be the basis of claims for risk factors, especially causal factors. Instead, their value is in providing information about the associations of outcomes with factors to enable another researcher to propose a sampling scheme (perhaps a two-stage prospective sample) that might be more cost-effective in future work, and to suggest which types of factors might be of the greatest interest in such a study. Enough examples exist in the research literature of false conclusions drawn from case-control studies (e.g., coffee drinking and pancreatic cancer) to warrant great caution in drawing any specific conclusions from case-control studies.

Phase II: Observational Longitudinal Studies Constitute Our Proposed Phase II of Risk Estimation

Again, finding examples of well-done longitudinal studies was easy. Picking which one to present was more challenging. First, there are fewer longitudinal studies—they are more difficult, are more expensive, and take longer to conduct. Second, and most important, the potential for design errors in a longitudinal study is much higher. At the end of a longitudinal study, often researchers will comment on what they would have done differently in the design, had they known what they learned over the course of the study. Longitudinal studies are simply more difficult to design, and paraphrasing a comment made by Light et al.,[3] "You can't fix by analysis what you screw up by design."

Longitudinal studies that are based on the results of well-done cross-sectional and/or case-control studies have a leg up in achieving a good design. The previous studies might suggest which populations to sample, how to access individuals in those populations, when in the life course should the study begin and end, and how frequently each individual should be observed. Phase I studies can also suggest which measures should be taken, when and how they should be taken, and how best to make the diagnoses. Phase I studies can also provide information for researchers to determine the most appropriate sample size for a phase II study.

Consider Example 13.2, which describes a well-designed longitudinal study.

EXAMPLE 13.2

Researchers studied the relationship between plasma homocysteine (an amino acid found in blood plasma) levels and congestive heart failure (CHF).[4] Previous observational and laboratory research (i.e., phase I studies) had suggested that elevated plasma homocysteine levels might be related to a higher risk of CHF.

This study included 2,491 adults (1,547 women and 944 men) who participated in the Framingham Heart Study during the 1979–1982 and 1986–1990 examinations. Participants were free of CHF and prior myocardial infarction at the start of the study (baseline) and were prospectively followed for an average of seven years, with assessments taken every two years.

Researchers analyzed men and women separately, as is customary and warranted in any heart disease study, since gender itself is a fixed marker for heart disease and may moderate the effect of other risk factors. The average age at baseline was 72.4 years for women and 71.6 years for men. Thus, the researchers wisely chose to start follow-up at an age where the risk of CHF is already high. Eighty-eight of the women (about 6%) and 68 of the men (about 7%) developed CHF during follow-up.

The research showed that both men and women above the median plasma homocysteine level for their age and gender group were more likely to be among the ones who developed CHF. Using survival analyses, the researchers demonstrated that plasma homocysteine level is a risk factor in older adults for subsequent CHF.

However, the research did not and could not show that plasma homocysteine level is a causal risk factor for CHF—this was, after all, simply an observational study. The researchers recognized and carefully spelled out this limitation in their results, saying that their findings "raise the possibility of a causal relation between increased plasma homocysteine levels and CHF," but also offering alternative explanations of why those who developed CHF may have had higher homocysteine levels without homocysteine level being a causal risk factor. Furthermore, the researchers concluded with the warning that more (phase II) studies like this one are required. They then recommend that if their findings are confirmed, randomized clinical trials (phase III) should follow to examine the possibility that lowering elevated homocysteine levels through vitamin therapy with folic acid, alone or in combination with pyridoxine hydrochloride and cyanocobalamin, may reduce the risk of CHF.

In contrast, consider Example 13.3, another equally well-designed study that used a different tone in their reporting. This particular study generated big and possibly misleading headlines.

EXAMPLE 13.3

Another recent and large longitudinal study[5] (404,576 men and 495,477 women) examined the relationship between body mass index (BMI) at baseline and subsequent death from cancer. Researchers followed participants starting in 1982 for about 16 years. The average age of participants at enrollment was 57 years. Hence, as above, follow-up began when the risk of the outcome was already quite high. BMI was based on self-report of height and weight at baseline. After 16 years of follow-up, 32,303 (about 8%) of men died of cancer and 24,842 (about 5%) of women died of cancer.

This study and the plasma homocysteine study of Example 13.2 had very similar designs and were analyzed using similar techniques (survival analysis). This study even had the advantage of a larger sample size and a longer follow-up. The differences, however, between these two studies emerge in the claims the researchers made in the reports. For example, authors of the BMI and cancer study wrote:

> On the basis of associations observed in this study, we estimate that current patterns of overweight and obesity in the United States could account for 14 percent of all deaths from cancer in men and 20 percent of those in women.[5(p1625)]

> Under the assumption that these relations are causal, the public health implications for the United States are profound: more than 90,000 deaths per year from cancer might be avoided if everyone in the adult population could maintain a body-mass index under 25.0 throughout life.[5(p1634)]

> From our results, we estimate that 90,000 deaths due to cancer could be prevented each year in the United States if men and women could maintain normal weight.[5(p1637)]

Although the phrases quoted in Example 13.3, "could account," "might be avoided," and "could be prevented," do not mean "does account," "will be avoided," and "will be prevented," the implications were that the researchers themselves were willing to assume that obesity is causal. The public media, not surprisingly, took the message from this study that obesity causes cancer with leading statements such as this one:

> Obesity plays a much bigger role in causing cancer than researchers had previously believed, accounting for 14 percent of cancers in men and 20 percent in women, according to a massive new study by the American Cancer Society.[6]

Such claims, whether made explicitly or, as here, by implication, will not even be tested until a randomized clinical trial in which, for example, individuals are randomly assigned to a treatment group aided to maintain ideal weight or a control group. Before that time, the researchers should have avoided any suggestion that obesity was causal, preferably even including a warning (like the one in Example 13.2) to the media and the public that such conclusions are premature.

Our point in presenting here two similarly well-designed studies in Examples 13.2 and 13.3 is to compare and contrast how the reporting of results can blur what part of the "story" a study is telling. The authors of the homocysteine and CHF study recognized and clearly stated the limits of their results; the authors of the obesity and cancer study did not do so quite so clearly. While no research groups can control how the media understand and report the finding, they must be as diligent as possible to avoid any indication of causality in reporting their results.

Phase III: The Final Phase of Risk Estimation Is the Randomized Clinical Trial

As in the drug approval process, the final phase of risk research we propose, prior to putting the result into practice, is a randomized clinical trial. The design of a randomized clinical trial should draw heavily on the results of prior cross-sectional and observational longitudinal studies (phases I and II) to achieve the best design using the least amount of money, time, and resources. Researchers face even more difficult challenges in designing a randomized clinical trial than in designing an observational longitudinal study, and even those studies that do have the three necessary components of a randomized clinical trial (randomization, blinding, and a control group) may have serious sampling or design issues. However, because the rules governing how such trials should be done are well and widely known, there are many randomized clinical trials that might be presented as an example.

Because it highlights so well the issues discussed here, the Women's Health Initiative randomized clinical trial studying hormone replacement therapy (HRT) serves as an excellent example. The Women's Health Initiative researchers dropped a bombshell in the summer of 2002 when they announced the early termination of part of their study because women in the treatment group taking the most common form of HRT had significantly more cases of breast cancer, strokes, heart attacks, and blood clots than did women taking a placebo.[7] Doctors were inundated with troubled calls from women who had been prescribed HRT, many for the purpose of preventing some of the very diseases—specifically heart disease—that researchers had found HRT actually promoted.

Phase I for this study was well established by numerous observational studies noting that the risk of coronary heart disease for women was distinctly lower than that for men up to the age of menopause, after which the rates for men and women tended to converge. That suggested the hypothesis that female hormones were protective against heart disease. Researchers also conducted several phase II studies, including both case-control studies and longitudinal observational studies. While some results conflicted, the general consensus, particularly after the influential Nurses' Health Study[8] (which we discussed in Example 6.6), was that HRT at or about the time of menopause was a protective risk factor against coronary heart disease. In addition, all these studies indicated that the incidence of heart disease was likely to be low in a short follow-up time and thus that any randomized clinical trial in phase III would have to be relatively long in duration and have a very large sample size. The stage was then set for a phase III study such as the Women's Health Initiative study on HRT, as described in Example 13.4.

EXAMPLE 13.4

Between 1993 and 1998, the Women's Health Initiative researchers enrolled 16,608 postmenopausal predominantly healthy women between the ages of 50 and 79 each with an intact uterus into this 40-site randomized clinical trial with a planned duration of 8.5 years (to end in 2005). Researchers randomly assigned participants either to an estrogen–progestin combination or to placebo.

Phase I and II studies indicated that use of HRT would be protective, with the increased risk of certain types of cancer outweighed by the decreased risk of heart disease. Nevertheless, the researchers designed the study to permit consideration of early termination of the study at particular interim points, should the evidence indicate that either group of the study was at significantly greater risk of serious illness than the other. At one of these interim points the Data Safety and Monitoring Board "concluded that the evidence for breast cancer harm, along with evidence for some increase in CHD [coronary heart disease], stroke and PE [pulmonary embolism], outweighed the evidence of benefit for fractures and possible benefit for colon cancer over the average 5.2-year follow-up period."[7(p325)] The study was stopped and the results reported in 2002.

Although the differences between the treatment and control groups in heart disease, stroke, and pulmonary embolisms were statistically significant, statistical significance does not necessarily translate to clinical significance. In fact, of the 8,506 women assigned to HRT, 231 (2.72%) were known to have died from any cause by April 30, 2002, compared to a very similar 218 (2.69%) of the 8,102 women assigned to placebo. This result must be interpreted with caution, since the follow-up time varied, although with randomization and blindness, the distribution of follow-up times was unlikely to differentiate the treatment and control groups. Moreover, the vital status of about 3.5% of both groups was unknown at that time, but again, randomization and blindness protect against major bias from these sources.

According to the study report, "Over 1 year, 10,000 women taking estrogen plus progestin compared with placebo might experience 7 more CHD events,"[7(p331)] meaning that the NNT per year is approximately 1,429. That is, 1,429 women would have to be treated with estrogen plus progestin for a year to have one more case of CHD (coronary heart disease) in the treated group than if all had been treated with placebo. If we consider all monitored outcomes (e.g., CHD, stroke, pulmonary embolism, invasive breast cancer, colorectal cancer, hip fracture), the study found 19 more events per year per 10,000 women, translating into an approximate NNT per year of 526.

Although clearly the results described in Example 13.4 suggest that taking estrogen plus progestin is a causal risk factor for the monitored outcomes, an NNT as large as 526 per year suggests that this causal risk factor is not very potent. Nevertheless, the implication of this and other such phase III studies appears to be that HRT should *not* be prescribed for prevention of heart disease. Whether it should be prescribed for short-term use for management of symptoms in that much smaller subgroup of women who suffer severe menopausal symptoms or longer term use for that subgroup of women at high risk of colorectal cancer or osteoporosis, or for other such applications, remains to be seen from further phase III studies on different, more selective populations designed more specifically to answer such questions.

Since according to our proposed phases of risk estimation, the Women's Health Initiative study completed the orderly process necessary to guide medical decision making, why the uproar when it was published? Why did a *New York Times* article appear titled "Hormone Studies: What Went Wrong?"

saying: "For nearly nine months, doctors and researchers have been struggling with an intractable problem: how could two large high-quality studies come to diametrically different conclusions about menopause, hormone therapy and heart disease?"[9] Our answer is very direct and simple: the two studies referred to (the Nurses' Health Study and the Women's Health Initiative) served two completely different purposes in the process of elucidating the relationship between HRT and heart disease. The Nurses' Health Study was a phase II study, from which it was inappropriate to draw any conclusions about causality. This study served as one of the bases of proposing, designing, and implementing the phase III studies exemplified by the Women's Health Initiative.

Problems arose because the Nurses' Health Study researchers themselves, the public media, drug companies and their representatives, treating physicians, and the general public misinterpreted the findings from that 1985 phase II study. The study reported that use of estrogen plus progestin was a protective risk factor against heart disease in this population of nurses. What many interpreted, however, was that estrogen plus progestin use protected against heart disease—that is, they mistakenly assumed estrogen plus progestin was a causal protective risk factor against heart disease. These misinterpretations led to many prescriptions of HRT over the next 15 years.

Moreover, the report may well have even delayed the initiation of phase III studies. The investigators of the Nurses' Health Study concluded: "These data support the hypothesis that the postmenopausal use of estrogen reduces the risk of severe coronary heart disease,"[8] and later that "[f]urther work is needed to define the optimal type, dose, and duration of postmenopausal hormone use and to determine whether to add progestins." Suppose instead they had said something more like the concluding statements concerning plasma homocysteine levels and CHF, described in Example 13.2, such as:

> [T]he relationship observed raises the possibility of a causal relation between HRT and heart disease. However, an alternative interpretation is that individuals who self-report use of HRT are less likely to develop heart disease whether or not they use HRT, perhaps due to greater attention to health issues or access to health care. Thus, the current results should not be interpreted as proving that use of HRT prevents heart disease.

Instead, the authors of the Nurses' Health Study ended with the comment: "The ethics and feasibility of conducting a clinical trial to obtain more definitive information should be considered carefully," a comment suggesting that it might be both unethical and not feasible to propose a randomized clinical trial.

Contrast that with the appeal described in Example 13.2 for subsequent randomized clinical trials.

Indeed, the long time span from the publication of the Nurses' Health Study (1985) to the initiation of the Women's Health Initiative (1993) and its conclusion (2002) may have been the result of the premature generalization of the results of the observational longitudinal studies coupled with the suggestion that randomized clinical trials might face ethical problems. Many simply accepted that the Nurses' Health Study established the effectiveness of HRT to prevent heart disease and proceeded accordingly, only later to be shocked by the results of the first major randomized clinical trial that contradicted these results.

The Women's Health Initiative is, of course, not the last word on the issue. The part of the Women's Health Initiative we are describing tested the most common form of HRT (estrogen plus progestin), but other formulations of HRT exist. Also, because the study did indicate an advantage in the HRT group for menopausal symptom control, hip fractures, and colorectal cancers, other investigators might elect to do randomized clinical trials in highly selected subpopulations of women, such as women considered at high risk for colorectal cancers or for osteoporosis, where the cost–benefit balance might shift.

With twenty-twenty hindsight, we can see where the research process investigating the link between certain forms of HRT and coronary heart disease, among other disorders, went wrong. The mistakes weren't as much in each individual study as they were in prematurely taking action before the final phase was completed or even started. One of the most unfortunate parts of this story is the delay between the phase II studies suggesting that HRT was protective against heart disease and the phase III study that suggested it did not. Nevertheless, HRT was not that potent of a risk factor for heart disease: the damage of so many women taking HRT may not be as bad as the media uproar made it out to be.

Conclusion and Summary

The strategy we propose for risk estimation is to recognize both the value and the limitations of the different types of studies that might be conducted to piece together the puzzle of what causes a particular disease or disorder. This strategy consists of three primary research phases—phase I consists of the preliminary cross-sectional and case-control studies, phase II consists of longitudinal observational studies, and phase III consist of randomized clinical trials. No phase should proceed before the previous one is accomplished, and no conclusions should be drawn in any phase beyond the scope of what the research in that stage is capable of supporting. When steps are skipped, pieces of the puzzle of what causes a disease may be forced into the wrong places, possibly harming those who use the results, but at least delaying progress to seeing the whole picture until someone discovers the misplaced pieces.

Not all research groups are qualified or capable of doing all the phases. Some researchers or research groups are best equipped to do cross-sectional studies or case-control studies, others longitudinal, and still others randomized clinical trials. Even if one group were capable of doing all the phases, we have to acknowledge the benefits of having independent research groups check and extend the findings of others. Nevertheless, above all, the necessity of passing the baton from one phase to the next typically by way of different researchers or research groups places a premium on what we urge is vital to changing the face of risk research: clear and correct communication.

14

Hope for the Future

From all we have said to this point, it should be clear there are no simple answers in medical risk research. At the very least, we need to agree on a common language and find some workable strategy on how to sort, digest, and analyze the massive amount of material generated on a daily basis about health, disease, and medical risk. Indeed, the level of confusion surrounding these health issues is dismaying, particularly given the massive investment we make, financial and otherwise, in biomedical research intended to improve our physical and mental health. Why are the designs of studies, the statistical tools to analyze the results, and the interpretation of the results not already sufficient to assure the accuracy of the conclusions? We have suggested that very few of the problems we have discussed, or the solutions we have proposed, are actually new and unknown to risk researchers. Nevertheless, researchers will still find it easier to continue to use and apply the easy but questionable techniques established by tradition than to adopt the new, unfamiliar, or more difficult ones required to get the right and the complete answers. As we look toward the future, how can we as individuals, physicians, policy makers, and researchers motivate change?

What we can guarantee is that within the next week or so, you will be greeted by the same type of headlines that drew you to reading this book in the first place. For example, during the week of May 27, 2004 (as we were completing this chapter), the following headline appeared in the *New York*

Times: "A Study Questions Blood-Test Results on Prostate Cancer."[1] This article was based on a study published in the *New England Journal of Medicine,*[2] reporting that as many as 15% of men with prostate-specific antigen (PSA) levels below 4.0 ng/ml—the agreed upon threshold above which doctors recommend a biopsy to see if cancer is present—had prostate cancer. Before this study was published, we had already included examples in this book about the very same debate concerning the PSA test and prostate cancer. In the intervening time, not only has the question of PSA testing not been resolved, but it is not clear if we are any closer to an answer. Worse yet, PSA testing is already part of routine medical practice even in absence of clear and unambiguous knowledge about whom it benefits and how much. This latest study only adds fuel to the fire.

Long before the 2004 study, many already questioned the value of the PSA test in detecting prostate cancer. For example, the incidence of prostate cancer was considerably higher in the United States, where PSA screening has been more intense than in the United Kingdom, but the mortality rate from prostate cancer was comparable between the two countries.[3] In addition, the lifetime risk of death from prostate cancer has been reported to be 3–4%, while the lifetime risk of diagnosis of the disease has been reported to be almost 17%, suggesting that many diagnosed prostate cancers may be "clinically unimportant."[2] But at the same time that many were already questioning the value of having men undergo biopsies when their PSA levels exceeded 4.0 ng/ml, television news stories reporting on this latest study posed the question of whether this threshold should be lowered.[4] Lowering this threshold would result in *more* men undergoing biopsies to detect *more* possibly clinically unimportant cancers. For this reason, the authors of this latest study do not suggest lowering the threshold, but what do their results suggest? Should doctors continue to give PSA tests, and if they do, to whom should they give them, and how should they respond to the results of the test?

These questions do not differ from the questions asked in the early 1990s when the PSA level was first beginning to be used as a screening tool to detect prostate cancer.[5] Studies continue, and we can only hope that they take a more direct path to answering the question of whether or not the PSA test is a valuable tool for detecting prostate cancer, and if it is not, what is. Ideally, we'd like to see a moderator–mediator analysis both to weed out unimportant risk factors and to determine how the important ones work together in predicting prostate cancer. Perhaps following such an analysis with building an ROC tree or some other "decision" tree may be more helpful in deciding how to juxtapose multiple risk factors to prevent death from prostate cancer without causing impotency and incontinence in men who would never have died from the disease.

We have outlined research strategies for sorting out at least some of these issues pertinent to the PSA and prostate cancer debate, while illustrating how many research studies already fit somewhere into this strategy. In fact, all we are arguing is that researchers recognize how each study fits into the big picture as well as recognize the limitations of each particular type of study. Some of the most important elements of strategies we propose here are actually quite simple. For example, if everyone adhered to strict scientific terminology and therefore didn't call—or even suggest—that a correlate might be a risk factor, that a risk factor with little potency matters, or that a risk factor not shown to be a causal risk factor is a cause, we might avoid at least some of the damaging reversals we have seen in risk research over the past few decades. Surely, asking that scientists be precise in their use of scientific language so that scientific communication does not mislead is little enough to ask!

If we could only get that done, then those who do cross-sectional studies or case-control studies would be obliged to report at most that they have documented correlates, not risk factors, and not causal risk factors. If scientists felt it important to document risk factors, they would be forced to do longitudinal studies; if they felt it important to document causal factors, they would be forced to do randomized clinical trials. Thus, even a slight shift toward a precise common language would repair many design and analysis problems that result from language ambiguity.

But of course we've asked for more. We've asked for well-designed studies based on reliable and valid measures and diagnoses. We've asked that statistical significance be augmented with close attention to clinical significance via reporting of potency measures. We've asked that evidence be amassed to document how risk factors work together. We've also suggested some methodological ways to answer these requests, but we also acknowledge that there may be other, perhaps better, perhaps yet undeveloped, methods of dealing with these issues. We also hope that we've emphasized that these methods do not necessarily need to be complex—in fact, to the contrary, the methods we present are quite simple and don't include complicated statistical modeling with many (or any) a priori assumptions about the underlying data.

The issue here is how this change can be accomplished, who will accomplish it, and how we will know it has been accomplished. We believe we all play a role in accomplishing this change.

Obviously, researchers are at the front line. Not only are they responsible for the quality of the studies they conduct; they also interpret their studies to the public media and thence to the general public, and they disseminate their results to their clinical and research colleagues. When a clinician makes a wrong decision in treating a patient, clearly the clinician knows that he or she bears some responsibility to rethink the decision and pursue another clinical course. Anything else would be unethical if not actual malpractice. But at most one patient is harmed with one decision. On the other hand, if that clinician is a clinical researcher and makes a wrong decision in disseminating the results of his or her study to colleagues, to the public media, and to the general public, that one wrong decision may harm many patients. Most clinical researchers are acutely conscious of this and take great care not to mislead, but there are enough examples where harm is done to consider the issue seriously.

When, some 15 years ago, the protective role of hormone replacement therapy (HRT) against heart disease took hold and was translated into clinical practice on the basis of cross-sectional, case-control, and observational longitudinal studies, why did the scientists who conducted these studies not warn, loud and clear, about the limitations of their studies? Why did they not point out that sampling and selection biases could account for many of their findings; that their analytic procedures were, in some cases, based on assumptions unlikely to be true in this population; that until randomized clinical trials were done, no one should draw causal inferences from their studies? Fifteen years down the line, and after many women were prescribed HRT with the suggestion that among its benefits was protection against heart disease, we hear scientists explaining why those original studies misled. But surely these same scientists knew 15 years ago that the features they now cite as explanations of erroneous conclusions were even then possible sources of error. It would be far better that scientists themselves point out the limitations of their own studies, to place their own studies in the appropriate context, than to wait for errors to be found by other scientists after the damage is done.

But consider also the message we have *not* heard loud and clear from the results of the Women's Health Initiative group, hard as they have tried. As we described in Example 13.4, the NNT of HRT as a risk factor for any of the negative outcomes monitored in the Women's Health Initiative study (e.g., heart disease, stroke, pulmonary embolism, invasive breast cancer, colorectal cancer, hip fracture, etc.) is approximately 526 per year. That is, about 526 women would have to be treated with the estrogen–progestin combination for a year to have one more death than if the same 526 women had been treated with placebo. The amount of concern, sometimes approaching panic, about the consequences of past use of HRT is perhaps misplaced, and at the same time, we may be losing sight of the benefits of HRT. The current researchers are pointing out that, while their study does establish that there is a causal effect of HRT on all-cause mortality, the size of this effect is very small.[6] However, this message is not highlighted in press coverage and may not have been heard by the thousands of women now attempting to get off

HRT. For the vast majority of women who took HRT, their survival time is likely not appreciably altered. If this message is also not emphasized, the pendulum may swing from the extreme where all menopausal women are encouraged to take HRT to the other extreme where all menopausal women are discouraged from HRT, even when it is truly needed.

Fortunately, the major protection against these problems in research, the peer review system for grant proposals and publication of results, is already in place. What if funders, editors, and the reviewers of submitted proposals and reports were to demand that researchers more carefully spell out how each proposed project fits with knowledge generated in past research and document that the design is appropriate to the phase of the research progress? Ideally, then cross-sectional and case-control studies would be approved only at the stage of knowledge when they are needed (phase I), longitudinal studies would be expedited (phase II), and inferences of cause would be allowed only when randomized clinical trials are done (phase III) or when the convergence of evidence is overwhelmingly convincing. Such a process would reduce wasted research dollars as well as save precious research time and, most important, avoid misleading results.

The problem is that those who are reviewers and editors are often themselves researchers who, in their own past research, have committed the same types of errors. That makes it hard to change—hard, but not impossible. All research is done using the knowledge available *at the time the study is proposed.* Any errors that have been committed in the past were assuredly not deliberately intended to mislead.

It would be an easy matter for readers to investigate the past research of the present authors and find many instances in which we, too, committed such errors. When many of the issues here discussed were first developed in meetings of the MacArthur Network on Psychopathology and Development, we were all actively involved in research in which we were doing many of the things that we now counsel against. Early in subsequent discussions, often one of us would cite a result as proving that something was a "c-c-caus . . . , uh, risk factor" or "r-r-risk- . . . , uh, correlate" for some outcome, with a furtive look around the table to verify that the term was being used correctly. Or begin to make a statement about a moderator, only to be forced to pause in order to recall exactly what was shown and mentally checking the list of requirements to see whether the term was used correctly. None of us was trained to use the risk language quite as precisely as we here describe; all of us have a long history of not using the language that precisely, and much of what we read in the literature uses the terminology quite casually. Eventually, correct use of terminology begins to come naturally, but it is not quick or easy.

Journalists and policy makers could improve the situation if they became more knowledgeable in the questions they ask of researchers. Certainly journalists should be careful not to overextend the researcher's message and to confer risk factor status or causality when, in fact, the scientists are saying loud and clear that these were *not* demonstrated. But journalists can take the matter one step further and ask less careful researchers the tough questions: "Professor, as I understand it, this is a case-control study. Are you sure there is no sampling bias that might explain the findings? Are you sure there is no retrospective reporting bias that can invalidate the results? You state that up to 40% of cases are due to this causal factor? Can you be sure of the inference of causality given that this is an observational study? In any case, what exactly does it mean when you say the attributable risk was 40%? Does that mean that if we removed this factor, 40% of the cases would not have occurred? In fact, if we removed this factor is it possible that the same number of cases would have occurred?" We are quite used to having reporters asking such tough questions of politicians and entertainers to make sure the public is well and correctly informed. Why cannot more of the journalists who cover science and medicine for the public media ask similarly tough questions of those reporting scientific results?

If they did, researchers would have the opportunity to state why their results are important and in what way their results advance the phase of risk research. They would then have the opportunity to clarify, for example, that much research is meant to guide future researchers interested in the problem, not yet to guide clinicians, policy makers, or the general public in their decision making. Such questions would also allow researchers to clarify the public health significance of their findings if their findings are at the stage of risk research ready to be considered by medical decision makers. In short, journalists might be very helpful in clarifying risk research and protecting the public against premature use, misinterpretation, and misuse of the findings of risk estimation.

All of us can exert pressure by demanding better and clearer information from the risk researchers, by simply recognizing and ignoring risk research that is not well done or whose results are exaggerated. We should demand measures of potency that make sense to us. We should expect information not only on individual risk factors but also on how these risk factors might overlap or work together and how to use multiple risk factors to understand whether each of us is truly at risk of a particular disease or disorder. We should insist that risk research be structured toward efforts to prevent or to ameliorate the disorders of interest. When a seriously misleading result is found, particularly if it is based on research projects funded with federal funds, there should be an independent investigation as to how the error occurred, not for the purposes of levying blame or exacting retribution, but for the purposes of preventing any further such occurrences.

We have already begun to see such changes take hold. A review of a sample of studies published in 2002 in psychiatry (not usually considered as advanced in epidemiological research as, e.g., heart disease or cancer) shows trends in the right direction.[7] Psychiatry researchers conducted few cross-sectional and case-control studies and several longitudinal studies with as much as 20 years of follow-up. "Lifetime prevalence," a statistic known to mislead psychiatric epidemiology, was rarely seen. Some studies continue to claim risk or causal factors on the basis of cross-sectional studies or to claim causality in a longitudinal observational study, but there are also reports that carefully explain why readers should not interpret their findings as indicating a causal relationship and setting out what they would see as necessary in the next phase of the research on the topic. We found one report that correctly identified a mediator.

Other recent changes include the development of many Web sites that help patients become more informed of both published and sometimes unpublished results of clinical trials.[8] These trends reflect the emphasis many place on evidence-based medicine. For example, the *British Medical Journal* has produced BMJ Best Treatments,[9] a Web site providing information to patients directly of the most recent studies as well as guidelines similar to ours on how to evaluate such information and use it to guide personal medical decision making, specifically with regard to treatments. In many cases, this Web site acknowledges that on the basis of the research actually done to date, sometimes no treatment may be the best treatment of all—a concept that goes against the grain of how doctors sometimes approach problems.

In addition, we have witnessed very recent examples of the media being more careful in light of some of the recent reversals, particularly with respect to HRT. A recent newspaper article titled "Heart Medicine May Fight Cancer"[10] describes how researchers are observing a protective effect of taking cholesterol-lowering pills (statins) on all types of cancer. After describing the evidence supporting the protective effect of statins on cancer, the journalist said: "However, experts have been misled by such data in the past. For instance, based on similar studies, doctors long believed that taking estrogen supplements after menopause would lower women's risk of heart attacks. A careful experiment eventually proved this wrong. . . ."

The overall goal of this book is *to encourage a dramatic shift in the course of risk research,* and we are optimistic that some of this shift may have already begun. We hope that, once applied, the ideas and approaches described in this book will continue to reduce the amount of research dollars wasted on less-than-optimal research and the amount of clinical resources wasted on testing for risk factors that remain to be confirmed by good science. We hope that these ideas will prevent policy from being enacted without careful consideration of research methods and interpretation. We repeat: the consequences of poor risk research are too vital to accept imprecise research methodology, terminology, or interpretation, particularly when the ultimate cost may be the shortened duration and diminished quality of human life.

Appendix

Mathematical Demonstrations

Below we provide mathematical demonstrations of specific items discussed in Chapter 9 for readers who wish to examine these items in more detail.

1. For random decision making, sensitivity equals one minus specificity (Se = Sp'). That is, factors equivalent to random decision making are located on the random ROC.

Suppose we randomly select Q% of the population to call "high risk" and $(1 - Q)$% to call "low risk." If P people actually have the outcome, then the percentage of people who we called "high risk" who will have the outcome is $P \cdot Q$ (i.e., % true positives). Since sensitivity is defined as the proportion of true positives divided by the prevalence of the outcome, the sensitivity is $P \cdot Q / P = Q$.

Likewise, the percentage of people who we call "low risk" who will not have the outcome (i.e., % true negatives) is $(1 - Q)(1 - P)$. Since specificity is the proportion of true negatives divided by $1 - P$, the specificity is $(1 - Q)(1 - P)/(1 - P) = (1 - Q)$. Thus, one minus specificity is also Q, so $\text{Se} = (1 - \text{Sp}) = Q$.

2. Any risk factor lies on a line parallel to the diagnosis line that intersects the random ROC at the point (Q, Q). When Q = P, the risk factor lies on the diagnosis line.

To show this, first let's describe the equation of the diagnosis line. The diagnosis line connects the points (P, P) to $(0, 1)$. The equation of this line is $\mathrm{Se} = (-P'/P)\cdot\mathrm{Sp}' + 1$, since the slope is $(P-1)/(P-0)$ and the intercept can be determined by plugging the point $(0, 1)$ into $\mathrm{Se} = (\text{slope})\cdot\mathrm{Sp}' + \text{intercept}$.

Now if we add up the first column of the 2×2 table (see Figure 9.2), we get $Q = A + C$. But $A = P\cdot\mathrm{Se}$ and $C = P' - D = P' - (P'\cdot\mathrm{Sp}) = P'\cdot\mathrm{Sp}'$. So, $Q = P\cdot\mathrm{Se} + P'\cdot\mathrm{Sp}'$.

We can then rewrite that equation to $\mathrm{Se} = Q/P - P'/(P\cdot\mathrm{Sp}')$, showing that every point in the ROC plane can be described as lying on a line parallel to the diagnosis line (i.e., the slope is $-P'/P$). This line crosses the random ROC when $\mathrm{Se} = \mathrm{Sp}'$. Substituting $\mathrm{Se} = \mathrm{Sp}'$ into the previous equation, we get $\mathrm{Sp}' = Q$, or equivalently, that line parallel to the diagnosis line crosses the random ROC when the sensitivity equals one minus the specificity equals Q—that is, at the point (Q, Q).

Since, by definition, the diagnosis line intersects the random ROC at the point (P, P), a risk factor with level $Q = P$ must lie on the diagnosis line.

3. The 2×2 table can be reconstructed using $\kappa(0)$, $\kappa(1)$, and P such that any other measure of potency can be calculated using these three values.

$Q = P\cdot\kappa(1)/[P\cdot\kappa(1) + P'\cdot\kappa(0)]$
$\mathrm{Se} = Q'\cdot\kappa(1) + Q$
$\mathrm{Sp} = Q\cdot\kappa(0) + Q'$
$A = P\cdot\mathrm{Se}$
$B = P\cdot\mathrm{Se}'$
$C = P'\cdot\mathrm{Sp}'$
$D = P'\cdot\mathrm{Sp}$

Glossary

The following terms are also defined in the individual chapters indicated.

Case-control sampling A sampling method in which researchers recruit two groups of people: those with the outcome (the "cases") and those without (the "controls"). Researchers compare various risk factors between the cases and controls to attempt to discover whether some are more prevalent in one group. Researchers often attempt to control the variation between individuals from each group by "matching" controls to cases based on preselected factors of interest (e.g., gender, race, age). (Chapter 6)

Causal risk factor A risk factor that can change and, when changed, has been shown to alter the risk of the outcome. (Chapter 3)

Clinically significant association An observed relationship that researchers demonstrate matters in some way to medical decision making. (Chapter 4)

Correlate A factor that is shown to be associated with an outcome within a population. (Chapter 2)

Cross-sectional study A study that examines the relationship between potential risk factors and outcomes in a span of time so short that neither the potential risk factors nor the outcomes are likely to change during the duration of the study. (Chapter 7)

Diagnosis line The line that connects the ideal point and the point (*P*, *P*) in the ROC plane, where *P* is the prevalence or incidence of the outcome. Any risk factor whose level is P must lie on the diagnosis line. Any risk factor whose level (Q) is other than P lies on a line parallel to the diagnosis line cutting the random ROC at the point (Q, Q). (Chapter 9)

False negative An individual who is incorrectly considered at low-risk for an outcome according to a risk factor (i.e., the individual gets the outcome). (Chapter 4)

False positive An individual who is incorrectly considered at high-risk for an outcome according to a risk factor (i.e., the individual does *not* get the outcome). (Chapter 4)

Fixed marker A risk factor that cannot change or be changed. (Chapter 3)

Ideal point The point in the upper left corner of the ROC plane where sensitivity is one (i.e., no false negatives) and specificity is one (i.e., no false positives). A risk factor at the ideal point perfectly predicts the outcome. (Chapter 9)

Incidence The risk of an outcome in which *onset* of the outcome occurs within a specified period of time. (Chapter 1)

Independent risk factors Conceptually, independent risk factors are two risk factors for the same outcome that operate independently of one another—having one risk factor doesn't make it more likely an individual will have the other, and having one risk factor doesn't change how the other might affect the outcome. Operationally, researchers identify independent risk factors by not being able to demonstrate that one of the other inter-actions exists. Specifically, risk factors for the same outcome within a population are independent if:

1. They are uncorrelated
2. They have no time precedence OR if they do have time precedence, within the subgroups of the preceding risk factor, the potency of the subsequent risk factor is the same

Independent risk factors should continue to be investigated separately. (Chapters 5 and 10)

Level of a risk factor The percentage of people classified as high-risk of a outcome by a particular risk factor. The level of a risk factor is usually denoted by Q. (Chapter 9)

Lifetime prevalence The risk of an outcome within an individual's lifetime. (Chapter 1)

Longitudinal risk study A risk estimation study in which researchers collect information from participants over a period of time. At the beginning of the study, all participants are outcome-free. During the follow-up period, researchers repeatedly assess potential risk factors as well as assess whether or not the outcome has occurred. (Chapter 7)

Mediator Conceptually, a mediator is a risk factor that explains how or why another risk factor affects the outcome. Operationally, a risk factor mediates another risk factor for the same outcome, if, in a particular population:

1. The two risk factors are correlated,
2. The mediator occurs after the other risk factor, and
3. When researchers attempt to use both risk factors to predict the outcome,

either both risk factors matter (partial mediation) or only the mediator matters (total mediation)

When a mediator is identified, further research should attempt to establish whether the path created by the risk factor and its mediator is causal or not. (Chapters 5 and 10)

Moderator Conceptually, a moderator is a risk factor that can be used to divide the population into groups such that within those groups, another risk factor for the same outcome operates differently. Operationally, a risk factor is a moderator within a pair of risk factors for the same outcome in a population if:

1. The two risk factors are uncorrelated
2. The moderator precedes the other risk factor
3. Within the subgroups defined by the moderator, the potency of the other risk factor is different

Further research should separately investigate within the subgroups defined by the moderator. (Chapters 5 and 10)

Naturalistic sampling A method by which researchers attempt to draw a representative sample. Researchers propose specific inclusion and exclusion criteria, recruit eligible persons, and obtain informed consent. (Chapter 6)

Number needed to treat/take (NNT) The number of people that must be selected from each of the "high-risk" and the "low-risk" groups such that we can expect the high-risk group to have one more occurrence of the outcome than the low-risk group. Mathematically, NNT = 1/[risk(high risk) – risk(low risk)]. By "risk(high risk)" or "risk(low risk)," we mean the probability that someone in the high- or low-risk groups will have the outcome. (Chapters 4 and 9)

Outcome A health-related event or condition. (Chapter 1)

Overlapping risk factors Conceptually, overlapping risk factors are risk factors for the same outcome that are partially or wholly redundant to each other—they either measure the same "thing" in different ways or they are simply two different names for the same "thing." Operationally, risk factors for the same outcome in a population are overlapping if:

1. They are correlated
2. Neither risk factor precedes the other
3. When researchers attempt to use both risk factors to predict the outcome, both risk factors matter

Overlapping risk factors should be combined to produce a more potent risk factor. (Chapters 5 and 10)

Population A group of people with particular common characteristics. (Chapter 1)

Potency How much better than random—and how much worse than perfect—a risk factor differentiates those who are at high risk for an outcome from those who are at low risk, taking into consideration relevant costs and benefits. (Chapter 4)

Prevalence The risk of an outcome in which a person experiences the outcome within a specified period of time, regardless of when the onset occurred. (Chapter 1)

Prospective sample A sample researchers draw to observe future characteristics, behaviors, or events. Typically researchers draw a prospective sample to conduct a longitudinal study. (Chapter 7)

Proxy risk factor A risk factor that is a risk factor for an outcome only because it is strongly associated with another, more relevant, risk factor. Operationally, a risk factor is proxy to a more relevant risk factor in a population for the same outcome if:

1. The two risk factors are correlated
2. Neither risk factor precedes the other or the more relevant risk factor precedes the proxy
3. When researchers attempt to use both risk factors to predict the outcome, only the more relevant risk factor matters

A proxy risk factor should be set aside. (Chapters 5 and 10)

Random ROC The diagonal line from the bottom left corner to the upper right corner of the ROC plane, where sensitivity equals one minus specificity. Points located on the random ROC correspond to random decision making. (Chapter 9)

Random sample A sample drawn from a population such that every member of the population has an equal chance of being included in the sample. (Chapter 6)

Randomized clinical trial (RCT) An experimental longitudinal study having the following three characteristics:

1. The trial includes both a treatment and a control group.
2. Researchers randomly assign study participants to the treatment or control group.
3. The participants and research staff are both "blinded" such that, as much as possible, neither the participants nor the research staff know who is in the control group and who is in the treatment group. (Chapter 7)

Recursive partitioning An iterative process of using risk factors to split a population into two groups, and then each group into two more groups until some stopping criterion has been met. (Chapter 11)

Reliability of a measurement/diagnosis The proportion of the variability of a measurement or diagnosis that is not due or random error or, alternatively, how well researchers can reproduce a measurement or diagnosis on repeated trials in a specified population. (Chapter 8)

Representative sample A sample drawn from a population such that the distributions of the relevant characteristics match those of the population of interest. (Chapter 6)

Retrospective sample A sample researchers draw to look at past characteristics, behaviors, or events. (Chapter 7)

Risk The probability of an outcome within a population. (Chapter 1)

Risk factor A correlate that is shown to precede the outcome. (Chapter 2)

ROC curve The upper boundary (or "convex hull") of a group of risk factors for the same outcome plotted in the ROC plane. Because they have better sensitivity and/or specificity, all risk factors or combinations of risk factors located on the ROC curve are more potent than any risk factors located below the ROC curve. (Chapter 9)

ROC plane A plot of the sensitivity of a risk factor against one minus its specificity. Plotting risk factors in the ROC plane allows us to look at points corresponding to different risk factors to visualize how they differ in potency. (Chapter 9)

ROC tree method A recursive partitioning method that uses the kappa coefficient to determine the next best risk factor to split on. In the ROC tree method, to split a node further (1) the node must have a large enough sample size and (2) the risks of the outcome for the two groups created by branching is statistically different from one another. The ROC tree method uses no pruning procedures. (Chapter 11)

Sensitivity (Se) In a particular population, the probability that someone who will have the outcome is classified as high risk. (Chapter 9)

Specificity (Sp) In a particular population, the probability that someone who will not have the outcome is classified as low risk. (Chapter 9)

Statistically significant association An observed relationship that researchers demonstrate is unlikely to be due to chance. (Chapter 4)

Study participants A group of people sampled from a particular population who participate in a study. (Chapter 1)

True negative An individual who is correctly considered at low-risk for an outcome according to a risk factor (i.e., the individual does *not* get the outcome). (Chapter 4)

True positive An individual who is correctly considered at high-risk for an outcome according to a risk factor (i.e., the individual gets the outcome). (Chapter 4)

Two-stage prospective sample A sample that researchers draw from a population in two stages and follow prospectively. In stage 1, researchers draw a naturalistic sample and collect information on specific risk factors of interest. In stage 2, researchers divide participants into groups ("strata") based upon the risk factors. Researchers then draw a random sample (of size determined by the researcher) from each stratum and follow each for a predetermined duration of time. (Chapter 6)

Validity of a measurement/diagnosis The proportion of the variability of a measurement or diagnosis that can be attributed to relevant information in a specified population, that is, how well in a specified population the measure or diagnosis represents the characteristic or disorder of interest. (Chapter 8)

Variable marker A risk factor that can change or be changed, but researchers have not (yet) shown that changing the risk factor alters the risk of the outcome. (Chapter 3)

Variable risk factor A risk factor that can change or be changed. (Chapter 3)

References

Introduction

1. Stampfer MJ, Willett WC, Colditz GA, Rosner B, Speizer FE, Hennekens CH. A prospective study of postmenopausal estrogen therapy and coronary heart disease. *N Engl J Med.* 1985;313:1044–1049.

2. Wilson P, Garrison R, Castelli W. Postmenopausal estrogen use, cigarette smoking, and cardiovascular morbidity in women over 50. The Framingham Study. *N Engl J Med.* 1985;313:1038–1043.

3. Writing Group for the Women's Health Initiative Investigators. Risks and benefits of estrogen plus progestin in healthy postmenopausal women. *JAMA.* 2002;288:321–333.

4. American Heart Association. Available at: *http://www.americanheart.org.* Accessed March 9, 2004.

5. Moore TJ. *Deadly Medicine: Why Tens of Thousands of Heart Patients Died in America's Worst Drug Disaster.* New York, NY: Simon & Schuster; 1995.

6. Silverman WA. *Where's the Evidence? Debates in Modern Medicine.* Oxford: Oxford University Press; 1998.

7. Kolata G. Breast cancer: mammography finds more tumors. Then the debate begins. *New York Times.* April 9, 2002. F5.

8. Kolata G. Prostate cancer: death rate shows a small drop. But is it treatment or testing? *New York Times.* April 9, 2002. F5.

9. Lynch A. Breast cancer linked to use of antibiotics. *San Jose Mercury News.* February 17, 2004. A1.

10. Last JM. *A Dictionary of Epidemiology.* New York, NY: Oxford University Press; 1995.

Chapter 1

1. Lloyd R. Metric mishap caused loss of NASA orbiter. Available at: *http://www.cnn.com/TECH/space/9909/30/mars.metric.02/.* Accessed March 17, 2004.

2. Study links sleeping to attention problems. *San Jose Mercury News.* March 26, 2002. 2E.

3. Kraemer H, Kazdin A, Offord D, Kessler R, Jensen P, Kupfer D. Coming to terms with the terms of risk. *Arch Gen Psychiatry.* 1997;54:337–343.

4. Recer P. Breast-cancer links to genes scrutinized. *San Jose Mercury News.* August 21, 2002. A10.

5. American Heart Association. *2002 Heart and Stroke Statistical Update.* Dallas, Tex: American Heart Association; 2002.

6. Cannon CP, Braunwald E, McCabe CH, Rader DJ, Rouleau JL, Belder R, Joyal SV, Hill KA, Pfeffer MA, Skene AM. Comparison of intensive and moderate lipid lowering with statins after acute coronary syndromes. *N Engl J Med.* 2004;350:1495–1504.

7. Kolata G. New conclusions on cholesterol. *New York Times.* March 9, 2004. A1.

8. Shibata A, Ma J, Whittemore AS. Prostate cancer incidence and mortality in the United States and the United Kingdom. *J Natl Cancer Inst.* 1998;90:1230–1231.

9. Kolata G. Breast cancer: mammography finds more tumors. Then the debate begins. *New York Times.* April 9, 2002. F5.

10. WrongDiagnosis.com. Prevalence and incidence of depression. Available at: *http://www.wrongdiagnosis.com/d/depression/prevalence.htm.* Accessed March 31, 2004.

11. Feuer EJ, Wun WL, Boring CC, Flanders WD, Timmel MJ, Tong T. The lifetime risk of developing breast cancer. *J Natl Cancer Inst.* 1993;85:892–897.

Chapter 2

1. Henderson M. Breast is best for better brains. *The Times.* August 22, 2001. Home News, p. 9.

2. Breast milk found to cut leukemia risk. *New York Times.* October 20, 1999.

3. Hotz RL. Adventurous toddlers score higher in IQ study. *San Jose Mercury News.* April 15, 2002. 5A.

4. Working moms' kids less ready for school. *San Jose Mercury News.* July 17, 2002.

5. Tanner L. TV may "rewire" children's brains. *Honolulu Advertiser.* April 5, 2004. A1, 5.

6. Bancroft J, Skrimshire A, Reynolds F, Simkin S, Smith J. Self-poisoning and self-injury in the Oxford area: epidemiological aspects 1969–73. *Br J Prev Soc Med.* 1975;29:170–175.

7. Hawton K. *Suicide and Attempted Suicide among Children and Adolescents.* Beverly Hills, Calif: Sage Publications; 1986.

8. Kreitman N, Schreiber M. Parasuicide in young Edinburgh women, 1968–1975. *Psychol Med.* 1979;9:469–479.

9. Wetzel JW. *Clinical Handbook of Depression.* New York, NY: Gardner Press; 1984.

10. Kraemer H, Kazdin A, Offord D, Kessler R, Jensen P, Kupfer D. Coming to terms with the terms of risk. *Arch Gen Psychiatry.* 1997;54:337–343.

11. Ostrov BF. Seeking clues on fertility's window. *San Jose Mercury News.* April 13, 2004. E1, 4.

12. Study links sleeping to attention problems. *San Jose Mercury News.* March 26, 2002. 2E.

13. Haney DQ. Exercise aids cancer recovery, study says. *San Jose Mercury News.* March 30, 2004. A1.

Chapter 3

1. Gould SJ. Curveball. In: Fraser S, ed. *The Bell Curve Wars: Race, Intelligence, and the Future of America.* New York, NY: Basic Books; 1995:11–22.

2. Churchgoers live longer, researchers find. *San Jose Mercury News.* March 27, 2002. 3B.

3. Bramlett MM, Mosher WD. Cohabitation, marriage, divorce, and remarriage in the United States. *Vital Health Stat.* 2002;23.

4. Christakis DA, Zimmerman FJ, DiGiuseppe DL, McCarty CA. Early television exposure and subsequent attentional problems in children. *Pediatrics.* 2004;113:708–713.

5. Tanner L. TV may "rewire"children's brains. *Honolulu Advertiser.* April 5, 2004. A1, 5.

6. Robinson TN. Reducing children's television viewing to prevent obesity. *JAMA.* 1999;282:1561–1567.

7. Vedantam S. Study links gene to violence in boys who have been abused. *San Jose Mercury News.* August 2, 2002. 8A.

8. Herrnstein RJ, Murray C. *The Bell Curve: Intelligence and Class Structure in American Life.* New York, NY: Free Press; 1994.

9. The Infant Health and Development Program. Enhancing the outcomes of low birth weight, premature infants: a multisite randomized trial. *JAMA.* 1990;263:3035–3042.

Chapter 4

1. Cross, M. The butterfly effect. February 27, 2001. Available at: *http://www.cmp.caltech.edu/~mcc/chaos_new/Lorenz.html.* Accessed July 14, 2004.

2. The Lipid Research Clinics Coronary Primary Prevention Trials results: I. Reduction in incidence of coronary heart disease. *JAMA.* 1984;251:351–364.

3. Study finds no link between breast cancer and the pill. *New York Times.* June 27, 2002.

4. Thompson IM, Pauler DK, Goodman PJ, Tangen CM, Lucia MS, Parnes HL, Minasian LM, Ford LG, Lippman SM, Crawford ED, Crowley JJ, Coltman CA Jr. Prevalence of prostate cancer among men with a prostate-specific antigen level ≤ 4.0 ng per milliliter. *N Engl J Med.* 2004;350:2239–2246.

5. Okie S. Study: breast-feeding reduces cancer. *San Jose Mercury News.* July 19, 2002. A1.

6. Writing Group for the Women's Health Initiative Investigators. Risks and benefits of estrogen plus progestin in healthy postmenopausal women. *JAMA.* 2002; 288:321–333.

Chapter 5

1. Shilts R. Nightsweats. In: *And the Band Played On.* New York, NY: St. Martin's Press; 1987:149–150.

2. Baron RM, Kenney DA. The moderator-mediator variable distinction in social psychological research: conceptual, strategic, and statistical considerations. *J Pers Soc Psychol.* 1986;51:1173–1182.

3. Kraemer HC, Stice E, Kazdin A, Offord D, Kupfer D. How do risk factors work together? Mediators, moderators, and independent, overlapping, and proxy risk factors. *Am J Psychiatry.* 2001;158:848–856.

4. South-Paul JE. Osteoporosis: Part I. Evaluation and assessment. *Am Fam Physician.* 2001;63:897–904, 908.

5. Churchgoers live longer, researchers find. *San Jose Mercury News.* March 27, 2002. 3B.

6. Vedantam S. Study links gene to violence in boys who have been abused. *San Jose Mercury News.* August 2, 2002. 8A.

7. Scully JM. Asian ailment: unfocused research in U.S. *San Jose Mercury News.* September 17, 2002. E1, 4.

8. Recer P. Breast-cancer study finds chemotherapy not for all. *San Jose Mercury News.* July 17, 2002. A5.

9. Rothman KJ, Greenland, S. *Modern Epidemiology.* Philadelphia, Penn: Lippincott Williams & Wilkins; 1998.

10. Shepherd C. News of the weird. *San Jose Mercury News.* August 24, 2002. A2.

11. Jugdaohsingh R, Anderson SH, Tucker KL, Elliott H, Kiel DP, Thompson RP, Powell JJ. Dietary silicon intake and absorption. *Am J Clin Nutr.* 2002;75:887–893.

12. Caspi A, McClay J, Moffitt TE, Mill J, Martin J, Craig IW, Taylor A, Poulton R. Role of genotype in the cycle of violence in maltreated children. *Science.* 2002; 297:851–854.

13. Agras WS, Walsh BT, Fairburn CG, Wilson GT, Kraemer HC. A multicenter

comparison of cognitive-behavioral therapy and interpersonal psychotherapy for bulimia nervosa. *Arch Gen Psychiatry.* 2000;57:4599–4466.

14. MTA Cooperative Group. Moderators and mediators of treatment response for children with attention-deficit/hyperactivity disorder. *Arch Gen Psychiatry.* 1999; 56:1088–1096.

15. The Research Unit on Pediatric Psychopharmacology Anxiety Study Group. Searching for moderators and mediators of pharmacological treatment effects in children and adolescents with anxiety disorders. *J Am Acad Child Adolesc Psychiatry.* 2003;42:13–21.

Chapter 6

1. A NISE project. Planning to err? Then do it as publicly as possible. Available at: *http://whyfiles.org/009poll/fiasco.html.* Accessed May 4, 2004.

2. Recer P. Breast-cancer links to genes scrutinized. *San Jose Mercury News.* August 21, 2002. A10.

3. Fleiss JL. *Statistical Methods for Rates and Proportions.* New York, NY: John Wiley & Sons; 1981.

4. Study links sleeping to attention problems. *San Jose Mercury News.* March 26, 2002. 2E.

5. MacMahon B, Yen S, Trichopoulos D, Warren K, Nardi G. Coffee and cancer of the pancreas. *N Engl J Med.* 1981;304:630–633.

6. Berkson J. Limitations of the application of fourfold table analysis to hospital data. *Biometrics Bull.* 1946;2:47–53.

7. Berkson J. The statistical study of association between smoking and lung cancer. *Proc Staff Meet Mayo Clin.* 1955;30:56–60.

8. Brown GW. Berkson fallacy revisited: spurious conclusions from patient surveys. *Am J Dis Child.* 1976;130:56–60.

9. Okie S. Breast cancer not tied to birth-control pills. *San Jose Mercury News.* June 27, 2002. A8.

10. Marchbanks PA, McDonald JA, Wilson HG, Folger SG, Mandel MG, Daling JR, Bernstein L, Malone KE, Ursin G, Strom BL, Norman SA, Wingo PA, Burkman RT, Berlin JA, Simon MS, Spirtas R, Weiss LK. Oral contraceptives and the risk of breast cancer. *N Engl J Med.* 2002;346:2025–2032.

11. Bickel PJ, Hammel EA, O'Connell JW. Sex bias in graduate admissions: data from Berkeley. *Science.* 1975;187:398–404.

12. Kraemer HC. Individual and ecological correlation in a general context: investigation of testosterone and orgasmic frequency in the human male. *Behav Sci.* 1978;23:67–72.

13. Hand DJ. Psychiatric examples of Simpson's paradox. *Br J Psychiatry.* 1979; 135:90–96.

14. Simpson EH. The interpretation of interaction in contingency tables. *J R Stat Soc Ser B.* 1951;13:238–241.

15. Humphreys K, Weisner C. Use of exclusion criteria in selecting research subjects and its effect on the generalizability of alcohol treatment outcome studies. *Am J Psychiatry.* 2000;157:588–594.

16. Stampfer MJ, Willett WC, Colditz GA, Rosner B, Speizer FE, Hennekens CH. A prospective study of postmenopausal estrogen therapy and coronary heart disease. *N Engl J Med.* 1985;313:1044–1049.

17. Spiegel D, Bloom JR, Kraemer HC, Gottheil E. Effect of psychosocial treatment on survival of patients with metastatis breast cancer. *Lancet.* 1989:888–891.

18. Kaplan EL, Meier P. Nonparametric estimation from incomplete observations. *J Am Stat Assoc.* 1958;53:457–481, 562–563.

19. Efron B. Logistic regression, survival analysis, and the Kaplan-Meier curve. *J Am Stat Assoc.* 1987;83:414–425.

Chapter 7

1. Bramlett MM, Mosher WD. Cohabitation, marriage, divorce, and remarriage in the United States. *Vital Health Stat.* 2002;23.

2. Rind B, Tromovitch P, Bauserman R. A meta-analytic examination of assumed properties of child sexual abuse using college samples. *Psychol Bull.* 1998;124:22–53.

3. Voldsgaard P, Schiffman J, Mednick S, Rodgers B, Christensen H, Bredkjaer S, Schulsinger F. Accuracy of retrospective reports of infections during pregnancy. *Int J Methods Psychiatr Res.* 2002;11:184–186.

4. Terman LM. *Encyclopedia Britannica* [book on CD-ROM]. Merriam Webster; 2000.

5. Gifted child. *Encyclopedia Britannica* [book on CD-ROM]. Merriam Webster; 2000.

6. Kraemer HC, Korner A, Thoman EB. Methodological considerations in evaluating the influence of drugs used during labor and delivery on the behavior of the newborn. *Dev Psychol.* 1972;6:128–134.

7. Fleiss JL. *The Design and Analysis of Clinical Experiments.* New York, NY: John Wiley & Sons, Inc.; 1999.

8. Meinert CL. *Clinical Trials: Design, Conduct, and Analysis.* New York, NY: Oxford University Press; 1986.

Chapter 8

1. Study reveals problems measuring kids' heights. *San Jose Mercury News.* May 18, 2004. E2.

2. Lipman TH, Hench KD, Benyi T, Delaune J, Gilluly KA, Johnson L, Johnson MG, McKnight-Menci H, Shorkey D, Shults J, Waite FL, Weber C. A multicentre randomised controlled trial of an intervention to improve the accuracy of linear growth measurement. *Arch Dis Child.* 2004;89:342–346.

3. Mathews AW. In debate over antidepressants, FDA weighted risk of false alarm. *Wall Street Journal.* May 25, 2004. A1.

4. Landis JR, Koch CG. The measurement of observer agreement for categorical data. *Biometrics.* 1977;33:153–174.

5. Jackson A, Pollock M, Graves J, Mahar M. Reliability and validity of bioelectrical impedance in determining body composition. *J Appl Physiol.* 1988;64:529–534.

6. Farmer ER, Gonin R, Hanna MP. Discordance in the histopathologic diagnosis of melanoma and melanocytic nevi between expert pathologists. *Hum Pathol.* 1996;27:528–531.

7. Whitby M, McLaws M-L, Collopy B, Looke DFL, Doidge S, Henderson B, Selvey L, Gardner G, Stackelroth J, Sartor A. Post-discharge surveillance: can patients reliably diagnose surgical wound infections? *J Hosp Infect.* 2002;52:155–160.

8. Maughan R. An evaluation of a bioelectrical impedance analyser for the estimation of body fat content. *Br J Sports Med.* 1993;27:63–66.

9. Muller M, Bosy-Westphal A, Kutzner D, Heller M. Metabolically active components of fat-free mass and resting energy expenditure in humans: recent lessons from imaging technologies. *Obes Rev.* 2002;3:113–122.

10. Martin A, Ross W, Drinkwater D, Clarys J. Prediction of body fat by skinfold caliper: assumptions and cadaver evidence. *Int J Obes.* 1985;9(suppl 1):31–39.

11. Dolan CM, Kraemer HC, Browner W, Ensrud K, Kelsey JL. Measures of body composition and anthropometry and rate of mortality in women of age 65 years and older. *Am J Epidemiol.* Submitted.

12. Dolan CM, Ensrud K, Kraemer HC, Kelsey JL. Measures of anthropometry as correlates of body fat estimated by bioelectrical impedance analysis in Caucasian women age 65 years and older. *Ann Epidemiol.* Submitted.

13. Brown W. Some experimental results in the correlation of mental abilities. *Br J Psychol.* 1910;3:296–322.

14. Spearman C. Correlation calculated from faulty data. *Br J Psychol.* 1910;3:271–295.

15. Noda AM, Kraemer HC, Yesavage JA, Periyakoil VS. How many raters are needed for a reliable diagnosis? *Int J Methods Psychiatr Res.* 2001;10:119–125.

16. Kraemer HC, Measelle JR, Ablow JC, Essex MJ, Boyce T, Kupfer DJ. A new approach to integrating data from multiple informants in psychiatric research: mixing and matching contexts and perspectives. *Am J Psychiatry.* 2003;160:1566–1577.

Chapter 9

1. Kraemer HC. *Evaluating Medical Tests.* Newbury Park, Calif: Sage Publications, Inc.; 1992.

2. The Infant Health and Development Program. Enhancing the outcomes of low birth weight, premature infants: a multisite randomized trial. *JAMA.* 1990; 263:3035–3042.

Chapter 10

1. Wilson PW, D'Agostino RB, Levy D, Belanger AM, Silbershatz H, Kannel WB. Prediction of coronary heart disease using risk factor categories. *Circulation.* 1998; 97:1837–1847.

2. The Infant Health and Development Program. Enhancing the outcomes of low birth weight, premature infants: a multisite randomized trial. *JAMA.* 1990; 263:3035–3042.

3. Scott DT, Bauer CR, Kraemer HC, Tyson JA. A neonatal health index for preterm infants. *Pediatr Res.* 1989;25:263 Abstract.

Chapter 11

1. The Infant Health and Development Program. Enhancing the outcomes of low birth weight, premature infants: a multisite randomized trial. *JAMA.* 1990; 263:3035–3042.

2. Breiman L, Friedman JH, Olshen RA, Stone CJ. *Classification and Regression Trees.* Monterey, Calif: Wadsworth & Brooks/Cole Advanced Books & Software; 1984.

3. Kraemer HC. *Evaluating Medical Tests.* Newbury Park, Calif: Sage Publications, Inc.; 1992.

4. Efron B. The efficiency of logistic regression compared to normal discriminant analysis. *J Am Stat Assoc.* 1975;70:892–898.

5. Efron B. Logistic regression, survival analysis, and the Kaplan-Meier curve. *J Am Stat Assoc.* 1987;83:414–425.

6. Kiernan M, Kraemer HC, Winkleby MA, King AC, Taylor CB. Do logistic regression and signal detection identify different subgroups at risk? Implications for the design of tailored interventions. *Psychol Methods.* 2001;6:35–48.

Chapter 12

1. Kraemer H, Kazdin A, Offord D, Kessler R, Jensen P, Kupfer D. Coming to terms with the terms of risk. *Arch Gen Psychiatry.* 1997;54:337–343.

2. Kraemer HC, Kazdin AE, Offord DR, Kessler RC, Jensen PS, Kupfer DJ. Measuring the potency of a risk factor for clinical or policy significance. *Psychol Methods.* 1999;4:257–271.

3. Kraemer HC. *Evaluating Medical Tests.* Newbury Park, Calif: Sage Publications, Inc.; 1992.

4. Kraemer HC, Stice E, Kazdin A, Kupfer D. How do risk factors work together? Mediators, moderators, and independent, overlapping and proxy risk factors. *Am J Psychiatry.* 2001;158:848–856.

5. Breiman L, Friedman JH, Olshen RA, Stone CJ. *Classification and Regression*

Trees. Monterey, Calif: Wadsworth & Brooks/Cole Advanced Books & Software; 1984.

Chapter 13

1. National Library of Medicine. Clinical trial phases. Available at: *http://www.nlm.nih.gov/services/ctphases.html.* Accessed April 28, 2003.

2. Brooks TL, Harris SK, Thrall JS, Woods ER. Association of adolescent risk behaviors with mental health symptoms in high school students. *J Adolesc Health.* 2002;31:240–246.

3. Light RJ, Singer JD, Willett JB. *By Design.* Cambridge, Mass: Harvard University Press; 1990.

4. Vasan RS, Beiser A, D'Agostino RB, Levy D, Selhub J, Jacques PF, Rosenberg IH, Wilson PW. Plasma homocysteine and risk for congestive heart failure in adults without prior myocardial infarction. *JAMA.* 2003;289:1251–1257.

5. Calle EC, Rodriguez C, Walker-Thurmond K, Thun MJ. Overweight, obesity and mortality from cancer in a prospectively studied cohort of U.S. adults. *N Engl J Med.* 2003;3348:1625–1638.

6. Maugh TH. Major study links obesity and cancer. *San Jose Mercury News.* April 24, 2003.

7. Writing Group for the Women's Health Initiative Investigators. Risks and benefits of estrogen plus progestin in healthy postmenopausal women. *JAMA.* 2002; 288:321–333.

8. Stampfer MJ, Willett WC, Colditz GA, Rosner B, Speizer FE, Hennekens CH. A prospective study of postmenopausal estrogen therapy and coronary heart disease. *N Engl J Med.* 1985;313:1044–1049.

9. Kolata G. Hormone studies: what went wrong? *New York Times.* April 22, 2003. F1.

Chapter 14

1. Kolata G. A study questions blood-test results on prostate cancer. *New York Times.* May 27, 2004. A1.

2. Thompson IM, Pauler DK, Goodman PJ, Tangen CM, Lucia MS, Parnes HL, Minasian LM, Ford LG, Lippman SM, Crawford ED, Crowley JJ, Coltman CA Jr. Prevalence of prostate cancer among men with a prostate-specific antigen level ≤ 4.0 ng per milliliter. *N Engl J Med.* 2004;350:2239–2246.

3. Shibata A, Ma J, Whittemore AS. Prostate cancer incidence and mortality in the United States and the United Kingdom. *J Natl Cancer Inst.* 1998;90:1230–1231.

4. Common prostate cancer test accurate? *KRON 4 News On-air and Online* [television]. Available at: *http://www.kron.com/global/story.asp?s=1898930.* Accessed May 26, 2004.

5. Kramer BS, Brown ML, Prorok PC, Potosky AL, Gohagan JK. Prostate cancer screening: what we know and what we need to know. *Ann Intern Med.* 1993;119:914–923.

6. Writing Group for the Women's Health Initiative Investigators. Risks and benefits of estrogen plus progestin in healthy postmenopausal women. *JAMA.* 2002;288:321–333.

7. Kraemer HC. Current concepts of risk in psychiatric disorders. *Curr Opin Psychiatry.* 2003;16:421–430.

8. Landro L. How to find the latest on results of clinical trials. *Wall Street Journal.* June 17, 2004.

9. BMJ. Best treatments. 2004. Available at: *http://www.besttreatments.co.uk/btuk/home.html.* Accessed July 16, 2004.

10. Haney DQ. Heart medicine may fight cancer. *San Jose Mercury News.* June 7, 2004. A3.

Index